WALKING OUT ON THE BOYS

WALKING OUT ON THE BOYS

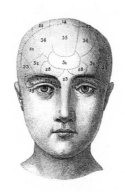

FRANCES K. CONLEY, M.D.

▼

FARRAR, STRAUS AND GIROUX / NEW YORK

Farrar, Straus and Giroux
19 Union Square West, New York 10003

Copyright © 1998 by Frances K. Conley
All rights reserved
Distributed in Canada by Douglas & McIntyre Ltd.
Printed in the United States of America
Designed by Abby Kagan
First edition, 1998

Library of Congress Cataloging-in-Publication Data
Conley, Frances K.
    Walking out on the boys / Frances K. Conley. — 1st ed.
        p.   cm.
    Includes bibliographical references.
    ISBN 0-374-28621-3 (alk. paper)
    1. Conley, Frances K.   2. Neurosurgeons—California—Biography.
3. Women surgeons—California—Biography.   4. Sex discrimination in
medicine.   I. Title.
RD592.9.C66A3   1998
617.4'8'092—dc21
    [B]   97-46561

FOR PHIL,

who shared these events with me;

and

MY PARENTS,

who molded my character

ACKNOWLEDGMENTS

This book would never have been written without encouragement and help from countless friends who were willing to read drafts of the manuscript, and provide honest, supportive, and sometimes painful, critique. Phil and I owe a debt of gratitude to all of them.

Special thanks go to those who really moved the project forward. Adrienne Rich and Frances Goldin saw promise in my ideas and awkward writing, and were willing to take a chance. Wonderful, supportive Sydelle Kramer slowly restructured the pieces of this story into a coherent whole, a process that forced her to endure more revisions than I care to remember. My intellectually gifted editor at Farrar, Straus and Giroux, Elisabeth Kallick Dyssegaard, ever so gently, but persuasively, applied the final veneer, and still managed to let me tell this story my way.

Finally, I can never sufficiently thank all those who were willing to provide unquestioned support, as well as much appreciated advice, during some emotional and distressing times. I believe they know who they are.

Frances K. Conley

While this is a true story and the real identities will be known within the Stanford community, some of the names have been changed so as not to involve those who were not part of the media coverage of events. The names of individuals who attracted media attention, top administrators, and the names of those who provided much appreciated counsel and legal help are real.

WALKING OUT ON THE BOYS

INTRODUCTION

Women have always played an integral, but subservient, role in the medical profession, primarily as nurses and technicians receiving orders from a male M.D. However, to the casual observer, in the 1990s, there has been a marked increase in the number of women who now function as physicians. Nevertheless, women must still struggle to gain admission to medical school, procure postgraduate residency training, actually establish a practice of medicine, and obtain faculty positions in medical schools.[1] And the fight for educational and occupational equality within a male-dominated world continues for today's female practitioners.

Elizabeth Blackwell is credited with being the first woman doctor to practice in the United States, after she received her M.D. from the University of Geneva in 1850. In 1964, a total of 758 women were admitted to medical schools across the United States, representing 8.4 percent of the entering class. During the

---

1 For an interesting book on the history of women in medicine, see M. R. Walsh, *Doctors Wanted: No Women Need Apply*. New Haven: Yale University Press, 1977.

1970s, as women enjoyed increasing opportunity and freedom in all facets of life, there was a rapid increase in both applications to medical school and the acceptance rate for women. By 1974, 20 percent of entering medical students were women. In 1984, the number had increased to 33 percent, and in 1994, to 42 percent.[2] It is estimated that by the year 2010, 30 percent of the nation's doctors will be women.

Medicine has perpetuated beliefs about its ideal demography and deserved elitism longer than any other profession. The academic arena is *the* place for a physician to build a national and international professional reputation; it is not in private practice. However, in 1993, only 8.6 percent of full professors teaching clinical medicine at medical schools were women, and the percentage change in this number over the preceding decade had failed to keep pace with the demographic shifts occurring in the doctor population which began in the early 1970s.[3] So the fact that much of the academic world is closed to women (and minorities) means medical school is and remains an institution of rigid hierarchies—almost an archetypal patriarchal society.

Academic medicine attracts highly intelligent, gifted people, but some are misfits—technically brilliant but emotionally insecure, even immature. Most enter the academy directly from fellowship or specialty training, without the opportunity to develop skills in human relationships that would come from exposure to private practice. Academicians have created their own language and discrete rites of passage suffused with a true mysticism and overarching arrogance. They are sustained by a system of exclusionary choice: future sons are cloned from the father. Anyone admitted is subjected to a closely guarded educational indoctrination, where the status quo is taught as the only "right way."

In the 1990s, many women, 45 percent of the total every year,

2 *AAMC Data Book*, "Statistical Information Related to Medical Education." AAMC, 2480 N Street, NW, Washington, D.C. 20037-1127, January 1995.
3 Ibid.

are endeavoring to shatter this system, accepting positions as assistant professors at a medical school. However, even these impressive numbers have failed to change things. Before the first promotion hurdle, women find they are working in a disinterested, disengaged environment where they are unwelcome strangers. Daily they confront the system's long-held traditional belief that the female sex is basically inferior.

Also, many career-minded women feel the need to delay the start of a family until they obtain their advanced degrees and finish postgraduate training; most men do not. Only recently have provisions for halting a tenure clock for maternity been instituted, and then not uniformly. The competitive, tenure-regulated environment of a university is not supportive of a simultaneous parental role (true for both men and women), especially given the time demands in a child's early years. So there has been a flood of female would-be medical academicians leaving the university to enter private practice, seeking more flexible hours and a balance among personal life, home, and career.

Reentry into academia once one has relinquished an academic appointment is virtually impossible. Thus, with women unable to establish a substantive niche, the old male guard of the university, accompanied by a carefully groomed new guard, continues to hold the power and make the decisions that rule the training environment of the medical professional. Women students may receive an education, but the reverberating circuitry of maleness in academic circles precludes their genuine inclusion in the total world of medicine.

For example, in 1993, women practicing surgery (including those in training) were only 6 percent of the entire surgical workforce. Out of a total of 4,526 neurosurgeons and neurosurgical residents in 1993, only 155, or 3.4 percent, were women.[4] While it is true that opportunities in surgery for women and minority physicians did expand in the 1980s (a response to both affirma-

4 Ibid.

tive action mandates and increasing numbers of female and minority graduates from medical school), in a new era of fiscal constraint and health maintenance organizations, where primary care doctors are needed as gatekeepers, and the number of specialty-trained physicians is being drastically reduced, the doors are closing once again.

It is medicine's rigidly controlled academic culture that precludes equal opportunity for all students. Women are still viewed as "not quite as good as," as well as "not quite as deserving of," and infinitely more suited to a career in primary care than in a surgical or medical specialty. In addition, we are continuing to educate our next generation of doctors in what can only be described as a sexist climate. In the early 1990s, surveys of female physicians revealed that 50–80 percent had experienced sexual harassment and/or gender discrimination during their time as students and residents—that is, when they were working in an academic setting. Male surgeons, uniformly, were the most frequent offenders.

My story takes place in one such academic environment: Stanford University School of Medicine. Stanford should have been different. After all, when Senator Leland Stanford and his wife, Jane Lathrop Stanford, executed the Founding Grant of the university in 1885 in memory of their only child, Leland Stanford, Jr., the senator described the university he envisioned: "I want, as far as possible, to have every useful calling taught and as near practical as may be, and I want particularly that females shall have equal advantages with males, and to have open to them every employment suitable to their sex." (I realize the senator's definition of "suitable" may well differ from mine!)

The university now serves as a temporary home for 14,000 undergraduate and graduate students engaged in many diverse disciplines. It has always been coeducational, but carefully so. During its first few years, 50 percent of the student body were women. But in 1899, six years after her husband's death, Mrs. Stanford limited the number, fearing the university would otherwise become known as a "female" institution. For the next thirty-four years, only 500 women were admitted per year to the freshman class. Ostensibly equal educational opportunity was extended to them. The school motto reads: "Die Luft der Freiheit weht"—the wind of freedom blows. An articulated university goal is that its motto apply equally to all regardless of gender, race, age, marital status, or sexual orientation.

Founded as Cooper Medical College, the medical school was originally located in San Francisco, finally moving to the Stanford campus in 1959. The newly constructed Palo Alto–Stanford University Hospital was opened the same year and was a joint enterprise between the university and Palo Alto until 1968, when Stanford bought out the city's interest. By the late 1980s two distinct tiers of physicians had evolved to serve the medical center clinics, the Stanford University Hospital and the teaching programs of the medical school. The academic structure remains the same now. Those on the more prestigious university tenure line are expected to develop a research enterprise in addition to teaching and, in clinical departments, caring for patients. Tenure—lifetime job security—is awarded after seven years to those who become internationally recognized in their respective disciplines. Denial of tenure terminates employment with the university. By contrast, physicians on the Medical Center clinical line are hired on the basis of programmatic need, to teach and provide patient care year-round, and, until full professorship, have faculty appointments governed by renewable term contracts. Among the criteria for reappointment or promotion in this line is the amount of revenue a given physician can generate. The trend has been to hire proportionally more male faculty into tenured positions and more female faculty into the clinical line. A substantial amount of research, as well as a considerable proportion of the basic clinical teaching of medical students in surgery, medicine, and psychiatry takes place at the nearby affiliated Veterans Administration Hospital (VA). Many physicians assigned to the VA for all or part of their tour of duty hold faculty appointments with the university in either the tenured or the Medical Center line.

Although the school of medicine employs the largest number of faculty of the university's seven schools, the size of its entering class is small—only 86 students are accepted per year. In 1991, 40 percent of the entering class were women (17 percent were targeted minorities). As it turns out, however, the structure of the professoriate is more important than the composition of the student body in establishing the prevailing tone. In 1991 only 9 percent of the full professors on the clinical faculty were women (there were no minority full professors). That in itself ensures that Leland and Jane Stanford's wish that women be educated to the same extent as men, and treated as their equals, remains unfulfilled.

I speak from personal experience. I was educated at Stanford, and I teach there. I am a tenured full professor of neurosurgery, and for thirty years have cared for patients in an academic medical setting. What follows is my story, one of many that could be told by women doctors across the country, about this institution and many others like it.

1

On May 22, 1991, I resigned my position as a tenured full professor of neurosurgery at Stanford University School of Medicine. At the time, it seemed the only realistic choice I had. In retrospect, I had little insight or knowledge then about the complex societal issues and academic power games that contributed to my decision. I was fifty years old, had been a faculty member with the school of medicine since 1975, and had many ties to Stanford's academic life and history. Stanford University has always been my home, as my father is an emeritus professor of geochemistry and I had grown up on campus. I also hold undergraduate, medical, and business school degrees from the university.

My saga really began thirty years before on a picture-perfect day of California sunshine in the fall of 1961, the day I matriculated at Stanford's medical school. I was not there as the result of a great deal of preplanning. For financial reasons, I had transferred to Stanford for my junior year (tuition was free to faculty children who qualified for admission). I had spent my first two undergraduate years at Bryn Mawr College in Philadelphia, an all-women's school. The time there had been liberating and exhilarating. I saw women as professors and student body presidents, women who sparkled with wit and intelligence and were highly motivated to do something important with their lives. At Bryn Mawr I learned I had the intelligence to do whatever I wanted in life. That lesson, unfortunately, was incomplete. The unfinished message was that intelligence and capability would not be enough. In addition, I would need to wage a lifelong battle to overcome imprinted cultural expectations, especially those defining a woman's limits, and be willing to persist in the face of misogynistic antagonism.

In contrast to my happy Bryn Mawr years, I was miserable during my junior year at Stanford. I felt I was back in bondage, tied by the same social constraints I had experienced in high school, where girls learn a fragmented self-image derived, in part, from the overt gaze of men assessing their desirability as females. At Stanford dating was more important than academic achievement, the only voices in class were resonant and deep, and career expectations for men and women students were very different. Early in my teenage years I had decided I wanted to be a doctor, not just a Mrs., although I certainly anticipated marriage as well. When I was young, our family doctor was a female general practitioner (unusual in those days) and I remember both awe and dread at visits to her office—it always had a strong antiseptic, sterile smell to it, and she was a bit aloof, and very intimidating. But, to a child, she exuded tremendous power reflected in pills, injections, pain, and soothing. Perhaps her example guided my unconscious career choice; I can think of no other reason for it.

But the undergraduate environment at Stanford was not supportive of women's professional development. A woman's intellectual life was not particularly important. Societal dogma held that women were not career-oriented, and would use their high-powered education as wives and mothers in order to provide intelligent companionship for a husband, and additionally, to nurture the next generation of boy children, imparting an intellectual advantage to *their* worldly endeavors. My dorm mates, all women in those days, gave in to this societal pressure, and would relive, week by week, their freshman year, a year in which, as "new girls on campus," they had a date, sometimes two or three, every weekend. Returning to campus as sophomores, or as upperclass undergraduates, they found themselves a used commodity with tired dreams, supplanted each year by the incoming group of brand-new, insouciant faces.

Not wanting to spend any more time than necessary in Stanford's stultifying undergraduate environment, with deliberate intent I applied for early admission to its medical school for the next academic year, and, fortuitously, was accepted, partly perhaps because my father was a prominent member of the Stanford community. In order to obtain my undergraduate degree I would complete my senior year and first year of medical studies concurrently. In the 1960s very few women were being admitted to medical schools. During the one and only interview I had I was asked if an application to the school of nursing might not be more appropriate. I told the interviewer, probably more bluntly than necessary, that I had more ambitious plans and had confidence in my ability to succeed.

An unusual number of women, twelve, joined sixty men to hear the dean's welcome on a warm Indian summer day in mid-September 1961. Medical school classes before and after mine had the more normal allotment of two to six women per class. We rapidly realized we would owe the profession a lifetime of undying gratitude for the gift of just being included. There were no people of color in my class, and I do not remember ever questioning why not.

Affirmative action had not yet been introduced to the medical profession, although in a few years it would become a major factor driving admission programs to increase much needed diversity in medical school enrollment. All of us were eager and ready to start a new, innovative five-year medical curriculum which was unique to Stanford, and a deviation from the standard four-year M.D. program offered by most other schools.

After a gentle day of orientation, medical instruction began harshly with gross anatomy. A home for the dissecting laboratories had not been included in the plans for the beautiful, new medical school, and this important component of medical education was taught where it had always been since the turn of the century, in an old, dingy two-story brick structure erected at a time when building codes for earthquake protection were unknown. The huge dissecting room on the first floor was permeated with death. Its atmosphere suggested that death did not require more sumptuous quarters, nor did those who worked with the dead. Even though another generation of young doctors would spend innumerable hours learning about the marvelous intricacies and secrets of the human body, a comfortable learning environment was not deemed to be particularly important.

Two parallel lines of wooden dissecting tables, each with a cadaver covered by a thick white plastic cover, were arranged along opposite walls in the large, poorly lighted room. The tables bore many scars and undoubtedly had seen more dead people over the years than most of us would in our entire professional lives. I, along with many of my classmates, had never before seen a deceased person, and I am not sure any of us relished the thought of spending the next ten weeks in an intimate relationship with a dead body. In some ways, removing the white shroud covering my assigned cadaver that first afternoon initiated an educational process of emotional separation from human suffering, where meaningful connectedness to another person became of secondary importance to the mind-numbing tasks of acquiring detailed knowledge and trying always to have the correct answer. Scientific knowledge and discovery have fueled our understanding of the body's machinery. We were taught great reverence for science, but little respect or empathy for the soul.

The rigid body under the cover was that of an elderly, overweight female partially wrapped in wet muslin. A tag with a number but no name was tied to the big toe of her right foot. Mottled discoloration decorated her back and buttocks where blood had settled after death before the embalming process forever fixed it in place. She had a distinctive, albeit somewhat distorted, face, and it was difficult to envision this body as ever having been a living, thinking person—someone carrying her own personal life's baggage of problems and joys. How had she died? Had death been unexpected? Had she worn glasses in order to see? Did she have cherished dreams that remained unfulfilled, tasks that she would like to have completed before her trip to eternity? And why had she chosen to donate her body to medical science, where medical students would inflict the final insults on that physical "container" which had housed and nurtured her spirit for so many years?

We little realized that first day how pervasive a companion the heavy smell and touch of greasy formaldehyde would become, earning it a permanent place in the memory bank of every physician. It was an odor and feel that not even a good hot shower and shampoo could erase. Or that we would become accustomed and oblivious to the fact that little bits of dead flesh would cling to our clothing and shoes, and entangle in our hair, traveling with us to other classes or even home, as if the dead were making a futile attempt to retain a tenuous tie to the living. It was all deliberately impersonal, a detachment that came from studying each organ or anatomical region as a separate entity rather than as part of a whole. We would find a similar detachment in later years of medical school, and in my career, when patients were anesthetized and draped for surgery. There, too, once asleep in suspended animation, patients lose their name, have no job, no cares, fears, no family, no love. They become the "hernia," or the "gallbladder," or the "brain tumor." For a few hours the surgical patient becomes an object, an area of surgical interest with pathology to correct. There is no need for humanity in these corners of medicine, and from the very beginning, we were carefully taught to disconnect emotionally from the dead flesh on the dissecting table, and subsequently from the patient in the operating suite.

And yet, occasionally, for brief moments, humanity would surface. A week after gross anatomy started, one dissecting team tied a yellow, helium-filled balloon to the toe of their cadaver. All of us were working at our assigned table when the anatomy professor entered the room. He was a slight, kindly man, his impassive face sculpted with deep furrows, who held himself very erect and had a demeanor which suggested a degree of resigned boredom from having taught the same unchanging discipline year after year to each new class of medical students. We all looked up, wondering what his reaction would be. After a quick glance around, he immediately went over to the cadaver-with-balloon and in a quiet voice that somehow was amplified in the sudden silence, so that all of us heard him, told the team that this person had been a friend of his—a good friend. He had been a scholar, a writer, a bon vivant, a person who requested he be allowed, with his death, to contribute to the education of others. All the professor asked, humbly, was that the students, all of us, honor that contribution appropriately. Head down, eyes on the floor, he quietly walked self-consciously from the room, away from our unanimous gaze, and when he returned ten minutes later, the balloon was gone and we were back at work.

Despite a knowledge revolution in biomedical science that began in the mid-1950s, I found the preclinical curriculum (the first three years of medical school) offered to us to be stylized, serious, and neither conducive nor receptive to imaginative thinking. Challenging "known" knowledge and "what would happen if?" games were not encouraged. Learning was rote, and students who memorized well tended to do well. We learned physiology, pharmacology, biochemistry, and pathology from the "normal" perspective of the 70-kilogram man, the paradigm upon which all traditional medical instruction was based, and still is, although to a slightly lesser extent.

We were taught that deviations from the male paradigm were, ipso facto, abnormal. Because they did not happen in the life of our normal hero, my classmates and I accepted without question the borderline pathology of women's reproductive functioning (almost the totality of "women's health" at that time), and we learned that only highly trained medical practitioners (mostly white men) could ease women through menstruation, pregnancy, and childbirth. Breasts of female cadavers were an unnecessary appendage summarily removed with rapid scalpel strokes in order to reveal the musculature of the anterior chest wall, which was then studied in intricate detail. I learned far more about the anatomical planes breached by a hernia than I ever did about the anatomy of the uterus, fallopian tubes, and ovaries. Middle-aged women beyond their childbearing years were not diseased, by and large, they were just depressed; menopause was an educational afterthought.

In a daring lecture session, sex between male homosexuals was discussed (twenty years before the AIDS epidemic began), although it was never graphically described and the act only alluded to by innuendo. And while we were taught that this certain aberrant behavior did, indeed, occur, it was, in the words of the male gynecology professor who discussed it, "yucky."

Most men, we were taught, only visited a doctor when they were genuinely ill. Men, but not women, died suddenly from heart attacks (actually, cardiac disease is also the number one cause of death in females, as was true of my cadaver) brought on primarily by the stress in their lives of unending, selfless work and no play, and wives who did not understand them. They also were plagued with prostatic hypertrophy and prostate cancer, and worse, some men even became impotent, a condition that merited a thorough investigation as to its cause and its possible reversal, almost regardless of the age of the sufferer. Men were thought to be more susceptible to lung cancer than women for unknown

reasons, and certainly died of the disease in far higher numbers—
it was just another of their excessive life's burdens. All my classmates, both male and female, blindly adopted the masculine orientation of our education—we did not know enough, or how, to
challenge it. After all, the medical world we wished to be part of
was one created by men—male professors, mostly male students,
and 70-kilogram male patients.

The linkage between smoking and lung cancer had not been
affirmed in the early 1960s. Smoking was even permitted in lecture halls when I was in medical school. Many days after lunch,
two of my more asinine, self-centered male classmates delighted
in smoking, not just cigarettes, but cigars, filling the close, non-
circulating air with thick, heavy swirls of foul tobacco smoke. I
find cigarette smoke abhorrent, but cigars are an abomination of
the devil. Pleas of physical illness—I learned and perfected the
art of programmed retching—and disgust from some of us
women (including one who was pregnant) were greeted with de-
risive laughter by the two smokers, who told us we had to think
and act like men if we wanted to be "real" doctors. I took anti-
histamines regularly during the first three years of medical school,
and unfortunately drowsed through more than one afternoon lecture.

Between my first and second year of medical school, I met Philip.
At the time I was not romantically involved with anyone. After
returning to Stanford, I had met and dated a steady beau, a well-
built gymnast and motorcycle aficionado. For two intense years
we had great times together at football games, the beach, and
fraternity parties, but pragmatically parted ways at graduation
(undergraduate degree for both of us) without much emotionality.
We had decided our futures were hopelessly incompatible. While
we had talked about marriage, I could not understand why anyone would voluntarily join the Marine Corps, and he could not
envision enduring four more years of all-consuming medical stud-

ies. A month after he left for Quantico, I literally ran into Phil, along with his javelins, on an athletic field at Stanford. I had watched the Russian women annihilate the Americans in the javelin competition at the U.S.A.–U.S.S.R. track meet in 1962, and decided it was an event I should try, even though I had never met any javelin throwers, much less held a javelin. So, with uncharacteristic bravado for me, I caught up with Phil as he was running warm-up laps, and breathlessly asked him, a total stranger, to teach me how to throw one. At the time he was an international track and field competitor who had represented the United States in the javelin at the 1956 Olympic Games in Melbourne. When we met he was still competitive in that heady world of true excellence few athletes ever attain. He is a very attractive man, and I was sure he already had a significant other. But I was not after him—I wanted to try throwing a javelin, which I thought was a beautiful event.

After earning a bachelor's degree in engineering from Caltech, Phil had finished his M.B.A. at Harvard and had moved West only a month before to join a small high-tech start-up company named Raychem. He was juggling his junior management position, requiring total dedication to a company trying to establish itself, with his own unfinished athletic dreams. Finding quality time to pursue the latter was difficult enough without distraction from a determined woman asking him to teach her. It was not love at first sight. Today Phil tells friends the attribute that cinched the relationship for him was my ability to do fifteen pull-ups "the hard way" (palms facing out, rather than in, on a chinning bar). I found I was not a great javelin thrower, but enjoyed trying.

As a second-year medical student I was not particularly interested in an amorous relationship which might jeopardize my goal of becoming a physician. However, our common bond of athleticism and similar educational backgrounds led to dates, martinis, lamb shoulder chops cooked on a tiny grill, and a diamond engagement ring. We were married the following summer in the backyard of the house I had grown up in on campus. I made my own wedding dress.

For most women, heterosexual marriage then represented a willingness to ally oneself with male power and patronage, and in 1963 I was happy to comply with this pervasive societal expectation. My conventional upbringing had always led me to believe that someone would be there to take care of me—and I had found him. It never occurred to me that in the future I might earn more than Phil did. Without second thought, I took his surname and fully intended to fulfill my obligations as a good corporate wife along with my medical studies. But marriage was also unsettling. Overnight, my identity changed. For twenty-three years I had been a Krauskopf. Now, suddenly, I was a Conley, but not a whole Conley—I was part of a Conley couple, and my individuality became subservient to our uniqueness as a couple, in which society defined Phil as "head of household."

However, ours was not destined to be a traditional family, even though I grew up in one. My father was always the "professor," the protected resident intellectual. My mother stayed home, raising her four children, until I reached high school. Then she returned to work as an educator and counselor for grades seven through nine. My mother wrote the checks and maintained the cohesion of the household, involving my father in the lives of his children even when he would rather have been reading about earthquakes and volcanoes. In general, in my family, men were responsible for gardening, garbage, and automobile maintenance. Cooking, cleaning, sewing, mending, and ironing were the feminine chores, although my siblings and I were cross-trained to an admirable extent. Education was extremely important to both my parents and all of us were expected to get a college degree. Beyond that, I was encouraged in my career choice, but not pushed. My sisters, a multilingual stewardess who flew with Pan Am for many years and a librarian/writer, as well as my brother, an architect, all married and produced the anticipated grandchildren, thus removing pressure on Phil and me from my family with regard to the next generation.

Many have described Phil as a six-foot-three Paul Newman look-alike, a most desirable bachelor who was ready for marriage and not interested in delaying his life's plans by waiting for me to finish medical school, even though my degree would irrevocably change the life he had envisioned for himself. Over the years marriage to Phil has given me legitimacy as a female who operates in a macho man's world. Those who would label me "emasculating" think twice about it after they encounter Phil. When we are together, the contrast between us makes me appear very feminine, an image I enjoy. I do not enjoy, however, being ignored, something that happens quite frequently when we function as a couple. Only rarely am I asked whether or not I work. At times at social affairs I am tempted to wear a T-shirt embossed with "I'm a brain surgeon—if interested, ask!" Physically imposing and handsome, Phil gets the attention, especially from women. In retrospect, we both agree Phil had no idea of what he was getting into when he answered, "I do."

Phil generously taught me life's perspective from the masculine viewpoint. He is an only child whose mother died when he was just a year old. Phil has no recollection of her, but keeps a portrait of a beautiful young woman with short, wavy dark hair, looking beyond the camera with a slight smile, on the top of his dresser. A picture of his father, in judicial robes, occupies the opposite side. Phil was raised by his father and, for a few years, his grandfather. When I met him, his father was presiding justice on the Fifth District Court of Appeals for the State of California, and had softened his male world with a late-life marriage to a remarkable woman, a Vassar graduate, whose very life educated Phil about strong women. Reflecting his frugal, all-male upbringing which lacked a consumer focus, Phil holds a tight rein on family finances, is a shrewd and careful shopper (always seeking bargains), a gourmet cook, and a lousy janitor.

Phil and I discussed and, without much thought, accepted the fact that my female classmates and I had to "let the boys be boys." Informal medical education taught an understanding of, if not appreciation for, dirty jokes and innuendo. To combat my total naiveté, I enlisted Phil's help and have him to thank for enriching my stunted virginal vocabulary. He even taught me the intricacies of games boys play—chugalug events, pissing contests, and lighting each other's farts with matches. In class, embarrassed girlish laughter joined the "hee-haws" of our male classmates when centerfolds appeared in the middle of medical lectures, ostensibly to add a wake-up jolt to otherwise uninspired didactic presentations. Augmentation mammoplasty had just been added to the medical armament in the 1960s. I reacted with skepticism when a plastic surgeon professor told us all women wanted the "really big ones"—every woman secretly fantasized about having breasts like Marilyn Monroe or Jayne Mansfield. The baggy implants (size: large) were passed around during class so we could feel how well they mimicked real, flesh-and-blood breast tissue. One of my classmates was teased unmercifully when his wife actually had a mammoplasty. He giggled with insincere embarrassment from the attention, and for many years delighted in photographing her and displaying pictures, on demand, of her scantily attired silicone cleavage. In medical school, however, little was said or taught about the psychology of a society raising girl children to believe their acceptance and success in life were dependent on the size and shape of their breasts.

Other vivid memories remain from the first years of medical school. In a small group session the male professor slapped the rump of one of my female classmates in a manner akin to spanking a naughty child, because she did not know the answer to his question. More often, as women, we were ignored, even if we had the right answer. While learning pathology by looking at slides of tissue, we were divided into groups of four. Three men joined me. One day as we were studying a slide, the professor dropped by our group and asked for our best guess of the diagnosis. After a couple of seconds I offered the correct answer. The professor looked at me and said, "Oh, I'm so very sorry. I didn't see you." The women in my class learned to deflect a few of the constant, almost daily insults, but we absorbed many more offensive slights that often had little to do with bad performance and everything to do with fortune of birth. We learned and accepted, without thought or any malice, the fact that most professors were congenitally deaf to the wavelength and decibel level of our female voices. Perhaps it also was difficult to hear us because every sentence we uttered ended with a question mark conveying uncertainty, even if none were there.

After three years of classroom and laboratory study we became clinical clerks and spent the last two years of medical school on the hospital wards and clinics in tutorial relationships. The pattern of the two years of clinical training remains the same today. Each medical student joins a health care team usually consisting of one or two residents, an intern or two, and an attending physician. The sick patient becomes the primary educational device, one's textbook, so to speak. One learns the art of taking a medical history, of doing a complete physical examination, and integrating those findings with the science of laboratory and radiology studies to arrive at the correct diagnosis. Once the diagnosis is confirmed, the team institutes what it hopes is appropriate therapy. The medical student or intern is the first to see each assigned patient, regardless of time of day or night, is expected to have the latest update on every patient's condition, the most recent laboratory values, and knowledge of the literature about each patient's disease. Lack of preparedness, or the wrong answer, is rewarded with ridicule, taunts, and ever more work, leading to a vicious cycle of severe sleep deprivation yet never being completely caught up. Once the cycle is established, the patient becomes the enemy, the doctor a wounded human being.

The training of a physician tends to be a demoralizing, dehumanizing process in which a medical student or young doctor is told, time and again, "you aren't good enough, don't know enough, and I (the professor) doubt you ever will have the requisite abilities to be successful." The intent is to spur the initiate to work even harder to gain knowledge and know-how. Most students do gracefully jump over this hurdle, and once over it, look back, vindicated, and, with a great deal of smugness, use the same harsh didactic techniques on those who follow, ensuring the perpetuation of a debasing learning process. However, women face a second hurdle, set close enough to the first, so that some never see it, let alone jump over it. We hear two messages: in addition to being ignorant, we are told we are also second-class citizens. Whether a woman develops into a confident medical professional depends to a great extent on whether she clears that second hurdle, or crashes into it, sprawling, spread-eagled, onto the track.

Doctors also are not taught to respect their patients. We teach doctors to "care for," as opposed to "care about," a patient, but, unlike the care rendered by nurses, an M.D.'s care is delivered from a position of power. The patient is an object with a disease that mystical medical knowledge and expertise can help or cure. The patient is weak; the doctor is strong. Can strength ever admire weakness? Genuinely empathize with weakness? Weak patients are sick twenty-four hours a day, seven days a week, 365 days a year, constantly sucking strength and energy from their physicians. If the patient had not fallen ill, all of us doctors and medical students could repair *our* wounded existences. Daily we try to regain balance in an effort to lose as little strength as possible from our lives, and live just like other human beings. Thus we attend to the unending chores of evaluating, admitting, and caring for patients as rapidly and expediently as possible, so we can sleep, eat, make love, or go to the bathroom. This life leaves almost no time or emotionality for humanity, for spending an extra five minutes just talking, or shedding a few shared tears with a patient over life's unequal burdens. Doctors are taught, above all else, and whether it be true, that they are strong, emotionally and physically, even when totally exhausted or sick themselves.

As women students, we were as well prepared as the men for the rigor of hospital work. However, we had not anticipated that we would also be dealing with horny residents, and the occasional horny attending physician. Woman as "fair game" was accepted as an integral part of the world of medicine—any woman: nurses, medical students, physical therapists, interns, residents, laboratory and radiology technicians, as well as the occasional female patient. Today it is still accepted. And some women need little in the way of coercion. The doctor is god, and every hospital is endowed with god groupies eager to satisfy sexual appetites in exchange for bragging rights—or a job, a promotion, or career advancement. Over the years I have received my fair share of initiating overtures. My wedding ring, or theirs, meant nothing. In the hospital, one-night stands, or prolonged affairs, are so easy. Call rooms have beds; many also confer privacy, as does the occasional linen closet, especially on the graveyard shift. Excuses to the spouse at home are glib and believable. "My services are needed at the hospital—I'm saving lives." How can such nobility be denied, or even questioned?

Once we reached this "hands-on" part of medical education—patient care—all students became conscious of a separation—never articulated, but openly practiced—between classmates based on gender. Because it was part of the medical system, it was sanctioned by the school, and in fact no one, including us women, viewed it as discrimination at all. The men learned they would become novitiates in a discipline of their choice, eventually ascending to a level of power and control where the work and servitude of less powerful others would not only accommodate their needs and desires but also build their very careers. The message heard by us women was that only a certain few disciplines were open to us, and that we should not expect a built-in support system. Dedicated career counselors steadfastly maneuvered us into pediatrics, psychiatry, pathology, general internal medicine, and family practice. My female classmates all complied.

When I started medical school, I had never envisioned pursuing a nontraditional career path. Early on I considered a career in psychiatry, perhaps in response to my mother, who, as a secondary school teacher, used her children as guinea pigs when she took a course in abnormal psychology and learned to administer psychological tests—on the four of us. But psychiatry in the 1960s seemed to consist primarily of treating drug-induced psychoses, and was a field where the practitioner had little apparent impact on a patient's life, or even mental health. It was not what I had in mind. I did not deliberately choose to buck the system and defy the status quo, but I was mesmerized, truly fascinated, by surgery.

During the first year of medical school I had signed up for an elective class called Introduction to Surgery, joining ten of my male classmates. They all thought there was a good chance they would choose surgery for their ultimate career. I took the class with no intention of going into surgery. I needed one more unit for graduation and thought the class would be interesting and not terribly demanding on my time. On the first day, the professor, who came to academic surgery from a military background, locked the door behind him after he entered the classroom, an unusual and dramatic move used to communicate that his class would start and end on time. After carefully inspecting his audience, his eyes returned to focus intently on me. He said slowly and deliberately, as if he and I were alone, "There are women who have finished surgical training, but there are *no* women surgeons." I scrunched into my padded folding chair, trying to make myself smaller, less obvious. But I was not about to get up and leave, not in front of him and all the others, brave unlocking that damn door, and give him the pleasure of a forced exit. After a long, very quiet pause for effect, the professor launched into his lecture on the surgical correction of hernias. I attended that class every week thereafter, mostly out of spite. The professor totally ignored my presence for the remainder of the quarter, his eyes always deftly skipping over my defiant gaze riveted on his face. I did receive my one unit of credit.

Thinking there was very little possibility I would, or could, go into surgery, I had taken the required surgical clerkship as my first clinical rotation, in order to get it out of the way. Unexpectedly, I fell in love with the bright lights of the operating theater, the world of sterile instruments, the drama of life and death, the actors—decisive, cool under pressure, with magic hands. Surgical clerks spend most of their time in an operating room at the end of a retractor holding organs and tissue back so the surgeon has a clear view of the pathology, and for long periods of time are unable to see anything but the surgeon's back. But there is an incision to close after the pathology has been corrected. Suturing surgical incisions on an anesthetized patient is where all doctors place and tie their first awkward stitches. I lived for cases to finish, tolerating hours of tedious boredom, knowing at the end I could usually cajole the surgeon into trading places with me. Positioned over the incision, my gloved hand would receive the slap of the loaded needle holder from the scrub nurse. It was such fun, and so very natural, perhaps from having learned needlework as a child.

A specialty that included surgery along with medicine was obstetrics-gynecology. In general, it was a happy discipline. Most patients I cared for were young and without complex medical problems. Out-of-wedlock teenaged pregnancy was a rarity, and most births were a joyous occasion for an involved couple. Men, however, were still infrequent visitors to the delivery suite. The presence of a "partner" did not become commonplace until the mid-1970s, a few years after heavy anesthetic sedation ceased being used. Four days before the end of my obstetrics-gynecology rotation, I helped a woman with Irish red hair deliver a beautiful baby girl. The baby's head was decorated with tufts of soft fiery red hair. I had talked with the mother-to-be after she was admitted in labor, and was distressed to learn that she really did not want her baby. It had been a mistake, she had a young son, and her husband did not want another child, but he especially did not want a girl. Their religion made abortion untenable. Moments after birth, I showed the baby to her mother, expecting that maternal instincts would overcome her negativity and she would reach for her child. Instead she began crying and turned her head away from her perfect creation. "My husband will never forgive me," she said through her tears. "He'll never love her as he does our son." I was stunned. Here, an intelligent, college-educated woman accepted, without question, the total dominance of her husband and his thinking over her, as well as the second-class citizenship of her new daughter within their family unit, and in the world.

I truly enjoyed obstetrics-gynecology, perhaps because, at the time, it covered almost the totality of women's health, and rotations on medicine, neurology, endocrinology, cardiology, anesthesiology, and radiology were fascinating, but all somehow lacked the quick decisive and mechanical aspects that I had found so enticing about surgery. I hated pediatrics. It was like practicing veterinary medicine. Most of the time the patient could tell you nothing, and each usually came with two highly anxious, irrational parents who detested medical students and would go berserk if I were sent to draw blood or start an intravenous line.

Gradually, as I found other clerkships to be less rewarding, I decided there was no compelling reason why I could not be a surgeon. Surgery excited me and I thought I had the aptitude to do it and do it well. I gave very little thought to the "surgeon personality" and whether mine would mesh appropriately with it—it was the discipline I was after and my choice was made without considering any future interface between me and the players who were already there. Once I articulated my plans for my future I began hearing from many well-meaning professors

not that I "could" not be a surgeon, but that I "should" not aspire
to be one.

For the national intern match in my last year of medical
school, I listed both surgical and medical programs, hoping the
former would prevail, but keeping backup options. I had decided
to try for a plastic surgery program, figuring it would be the most
receptive surgical discipline within which to defy the traditional
tenet that "a woman cannot be a surgeon." I matched in plastic
surgery at Stanford, primarily because I was known as having
sufficient stamina to endure three years of general surgery, which
is part of the required training for ultimate board certification as
a plastic surgeon.

After five years of medical studies and hospital training nine
of the twelve women in my class graduated in company of forty-
six of the sixty men. Four of the women headed for careers in
internal medicine, two in psychiatry, and one each in pediatrics
and pathology. All but one of us married. One of my female
classmates was married to a truck driver and already had five
children when she had started medical school. She seemed a very
unlikely candidate for medical training. Quiet, reserved, resource-
ful, always guarded, she headed for a residency in psychiatry and
eventually established a successful private practice. Another class-
mate conceived and gave birth to three children before graduation
and ultimately became a hematology professor at Stanford. Three
women married male classmates, and all of these marriages eventually failed. Because of our relatively large number, none of us
women had been viewed as being unique, so having to play a role
as the "first and only" was never an issue during medical school.

The school had originally expected to graduate seventy-two
identically oriented intellectual (as opposed to physical) physician
packages, leaving each of us to determine our future "fit" within
medicine. But in our world, "physician" was equivalent to
"male" and the identity transfer from student to medical professional was difficult for women. We had worked hard for our

M.D. degrees and in the process had really been forced to view ourselves as doctors first and females second. Identity as a woman was buried under our starched white lab coats, although the ability to care for women, as well as men, was not. I believe most of my class, both men and women, as beginning physicians, found caring for male patients more comfortable—they were a known commodity with defined health problems. By contrast, women patients seemed terribly complicated, because beyond childbirth so little was known then about their medical conditions and needs.

While I was friendly with my eight female classmates, we never formed true collegial relationships. We never learned to work together and support each other. I have maintained no contact with any of them outside of class reunions. Through subtle, unconscious social pressure, it seemed more important to be regarded as "one of the boys" than to be seen running around with a bunch of women.

After graduating from medical school in 1966, I started a rotating surgical internship—the first female to do so at Stanford University Hospital. As with acceptance to medical school, I was so happy to just be included I would have walked on my hands for the entire year if that was what it took to belong and be a part of this exclusive group. Although I was required to live at the hospital every other night during my first two years of surgical training, there were no on-call quarters for a woman surgeon. When the hospital had been built in 1959, the surgeons' on-call room consisted of bunk beds, dormitory style, for men only. Seven years later the head nurse on the orthopedic floor discovered I was trying to get a precious few hours of sleep, in between the almost constant nighttime phone calls, curled up on a tiny, short couch in a room used during the day for grieving relatives. Like a mother hen clucking over her helpless chick, she insisted on rolling a hospital bed into her cast room, next to a wall phone, and there I spent most on-call nights during my intern year.

In a passive-aggressive way, nurses can make life very difficult for an intern. Alternatively, if they admire and like an intern they can be of incredible help during that arduous first year. I have always had a decent rapport with nursing staffs, although not all women doctors have been as fortunate. Nurses endure arrogance and abuse from male physicians as part of their job; they do not expect, or tolerate, the same behavior from female physicians. I find nurses enjoy being part of the decision process and appreciate being thanked for their efforts on behalf of my patients. Being married also helped in my relations with nurses. Most enter nursing school with the genuine altruistic desire to "help people," but some also harbor a defined, or subconscious, ulterior motive of landing a physician as a mate. I presented no threat to any with such personal matrimonial ambitions.

It is obvious to anyone visiting a hospital that women have always been an integral part of the medical profession, although, until very recently, not frequently as doctors. The majority of women still participate in very defined, subordinate roles. If every female nurse, technician, and hospital housekeeper in this country were to go on strike, modern medicine in the United States would come to an abrupt halt. In the late 1800s women were thought incapable of practicing medicine; they had more need for medical care than ability to provide it. Medical training was considered too rigorous for the frail woman who was defined more by her uterus than by her brain. Exclusionary tenets denying admission of women to medical school never took into account the fact that nurses (women) worked long, brutal, physically punishing hours day in and day out, despite being burdened with the same biology of "temporary insanity" as those women wishing to be doctors. Thus, nurses became a subservient convenience, an essential part of that medical world established by men for the comfort of men. They were carefully taught to regard the doctor as a demigod, all-powerful, all-knowing, someone who could demand and expect perfect obedience.

Nurses' education and training, however, while rigorous, lacks the inhumane qualities inherent in the education of a physician. Even though required to do ugly things to a patient's body, such as giving enemas, inserting urinary catheters, or injecting often painful substances into flesh, they learn to deliver compassion and care when performing their duties. Unlike doctors, nurses *are* taught to respect their patients and are regarded by many as "angels of mercy" as they attend to chores others would shy from (such as cleaning up a large volume of incontinent, odoriferous stool or vomitus laced with blood and stale alcohol) in order to maximize a patient's comfort. Certainly their ministrations on an intimate level, where the dignity of a patient is preserved at all costs, stand in stark contrast to the aloofness of the physician. While making quick rounds, an M.D. usually stands at the foot of a hospital bed, staring down at a patient who, in more ways than one, is already down.

As an intern, the hospital became my entire world and any semblance to a normal married life for Phil and me disappeared completely. I was assigned to the orthopedic service at the time of our third wedding anniversary. Around 4 p.m. I finished helping a private orthopedist in the operating room but found six new patients to admit when I returned to the ward. And this was my night off! I dragged home, dead tired, at 11 p.m., having completely forgotten the significance of the day. Phil was sitting, hips slouched forward, on the sofa in our small apartment, his head on the rounded back of the couch, neck extended, mouth open, softly snoring. A warm bottle of champagne, unopened, and two empty fluted glasses were on the coffee table at his knees.

For survival Phil developed his own independent life with friends, social activities, and his own time clock. I spent much more time at the hospital than with him, felt guilty for doing so, but was powerless to change anything about this unyielding and unforgiving system. When I could join him in a scheduled activity, I did, but if I were "on call" he went by himself, and usually had a good time. I was not very good company anyway. Many times I fell asleep during dinner or even while conversing with guests. Phil has always kept scrapbooks about his and our life. The contents of these bound collections include snapshots, stubs of theater tickets, announcements for athletic events we attended, newspaper clippings, and pertinent portions of letters from friends. I am almost completely absent from the pages of scrapbooks covering the first two years of my career.

Phil expressed considerable resentment over the demands on my time and, either as retaliation or in desperation, established close and enduring friendships with a few women from his own work environment. This was not the happiest or closest time for us in our marriage—I did not know what to think about these relationships, and struggled to find a proper balance between work, which I loved, and the man whom I also loved. At the time I was quite confused, but probably should not have been so concerned. Phil had not had much contact with females as he was growing up, and unconsciously sought intellectual bonds with women in order to learn more about them. Over the years of our long marriage I have found that Phil truly enjoys a mentoring role (athletics, personal finance and taxation, wine appreciation, in-laws), adding richness and discovery to his own life through close interaction with carefully chosen others—both women and men. We are a great team and our marriage has survived despite our peculiar lives. Although social and gregarious when he wants to be, Phil learned, during our early years together, not only to savor but also to require long periods of hermitlike solitude as insulation against constant on-call interruptions to our two-person family peace—a trait that persists today. Weekends, on my "off" time, we began running together—first one mile, then two, progressing to six, ten, and more—finding comfort in each other's company and reduction of life's emotional stress in the physical activity.

When Phil and I have not seen each other for a few days, in a pattern that evolved from those first years, our next conversation is a recitation of what he has done in my absence. The world of medicine remains sealed within the walls of the hospital, unless I have lost a patient unexpectedly and need to share my frustration and grief. Early on I recognized an overpowering need to separate my world at home from that of the hospital. Phil has never been particularly curious about my daily patient care activities, and has never watched me operate. However, once I began working as an intern an important priority shift occurred in our relationship—the patient, not Phil, was now number one. It was as if medicine had become, not a mistress, but my demanding child, and as many new fathers find, that child was very hard on Phil's ego. One evening after I was called back to the hospital, Phil angrily burst out, "Why do *you* have to go?" I told him the patient was someone's father, and I was obligated to help him however I could. Adoring his own dad, Phil finally saw the patient as a person in a relationship with another, and slowly began to understand my life, its priorities and pressures. Understanding it did not mean he had to like it.

One day I was assigned to scrub with an old, revered, private general surgeon who was scheduled to perform a radical mastectomy, the only accepted therapy for breast cancer in those days. Community physicians have always participated in the teaching programs of the medical school in exchange for house staff coverage at night for their patients. While anesthesia was being induced, I introduced myself as his assistant for the case. Nonverbal communication in an operating room is with the eyes. The surgeon's eyes communicated shock, maybe even disgust, at my presence in his operating room. While I did scrub, I was not allowed to touch instruments or the patient, hold a retractor, nothing. Fortunately, I could learn by just watching, as the surgeon was a masterful technician. His experienced hands deftly separated the breast and lymphatic tissue from the muscles of the anterior chest wall. I winced as a portion of the patient's femininity was callously plopped into a stainless-steel bowl. The breast, resting in thin bloody fluid flecked with round fat globules, had landed nipple-side up, defiantly, like an accusatory eye, as if to say, "How could you? I, who have been loved and caressed, and fed the next generation, deserve better." The cancer was not visible. A pathologist rapidly left the room with the steel bowl and its contents. During the entire case the surgeon did not talk to me, but kept looking up from the surgical field as he worked, hoping I was but an apparition that miraculously would disappear, as the breast had, if he glanced at it often enough. Following the case, with his surgical mask still tied in place covering his face, he quickly retreated into the doctors' (read "male") dressing room, where he could escape. Women students have similar experiences today, although the surgeon is usually more subtle.

Women surgeons have always changed into their scrub clothes with nurses, in what used to be called the nurses' dressing room. At Stanford, during my training, this was a tiny, impersonal room invariably crowded with too many bodies and containing too few lockers to accommodate everyone. I did not have an assigned locker, hung my clothes on a hanger if I could find one, and kept all other valuables in my car. In contrast, the doctors, dressing room was a huge lounge, complete with an overabundance of lockers, along with recliner chairs, the latest magazines, and soothing music. Some years ago a female medical student, on the first day of her surgery rotation at another medical school, was led to the nurses' dressing room to change. She refused, stating she was training to become a doctor, not a nurse. Head held high, she entered the doctors' dressing room and proceeded to disrobe in front of some male faculty surgeons. Her dean asked her to pay him a visit the next day for a frank discussion about her inappropriate behavior. But slowly, hospitals, including Stanford, have changed signs to the operating room dressing areas to "Men" and "Women" in order to reduce the stereotype that only men are doctors and that all nurses are female. When new operating rooms were built at Stanford in 1987, the dressing areas for men and women were equal in size, and a lounge was added for the use of all operating room personnel. However, much informal discussion about cases, both pre-and postoperative, still takes place in the dressing area, and women surgery interns and residents are distinctly disadvantaged by missing this component of informal education.

As an intern I do not remember being at all concerned or inconvenienced by comments and actions that set me apart from the rest of the group. I shrugged off a series of lewd remarks and jokes precipitated by my having to share sleeping quarters in the emergency room for a month with a fellow male surgical intern. In the operating room, I did not consider having my neck massaged or kissed while scrubbing, the friendly arm draped across my shoulders, the playful tickling of my rib cage as anything other than innocent affection. I put up with all of it. I wanted these people from this strange world to like me, to be my friends, to welcome me into their professional world. Depending on the individual and the type and degree of physical contact, sometimes the attention was welcome, sometimes not. Inherent in a doctor's professional degree is the right and expectation that hands will be placed physically on another's body, sometimes on very intimate parts of another's body. In the doctor-patient relationship, the patient has deferred to the physician's capability and knowledge, and in so doing tacitly approves of being touched by another. It is a power play where the doctor holds all of the power. Some doctors, however, forget that the permission to touch does not necessarily extend to co-workers or peers. They touch indiscriminately to the point where it becomes a part of their basic

personality. Had I given it any thought, I would have been attuned to the power elements in many episodes of touching I experienced, and recognized them as the belittling, controlling
gestures they were. But none of the women in my world (nurses,
for the most part) ever made an issue of this touchy-feely, flirtatious, and at times not very attractive behavior, and I certainly
was not willing to call attention to myself by doing so. Besides,
chronic fatigue precluded thinking about power and power relationships. The only energy I had for thinking went to patient care
and getting the job done. I had learned to keep up and was having
a fine time as a member of our exclusive surgical intern group.

Every few months the Department of Surgery hosted a dinner
for the house staff (spouses not invited, so it was an all-male-
plus-me gathering) at a local restaurant—a gratuitous "thank
you" for our unending hard work. Liquor flowed freely, many
resident, staff, and faculty physicians would drink to excess, and
occasionally the restaurant would get trashed. On one occasion,
two residents played "dropkick," one by one, with a stack of
dirty restaurant dinner plates, splattering shards of broken ce-
ramic toward a huddle of terrified waitresses. One of the women
had sinned by not accepting the advances of a drunken resident
surgeon, and this was the doctor's way of getting even. Having
drunk more than was good for me, I thought it hilarious, and
giggled nonstop, experiencing exhilaration from the wanton, destructive behavior that would have been shocking to me, and others, had we been sober. There was an amazing freedom in having
the balls (literally!) to act out that way. I do not believe any of
the physician participants or spectators that evening felt the actions were deliberately cruel. Outrageous, yes, but not meanspir-
ited. After all, outrageous behavior was a God-given right for this
group of men—not just men, but surgeons, the elite of the medical world. And boys will always be boys. It never occurred to
me to join or even protect the frightened women.

All of us were lucky to have returned to home or hospital in
one piece after some wild, wake-the-town-up drives down El

Camino Real. I realized this medical world was as it was, and I could take it or leave it. Impulsive, at times antisocial behavior was an integral part of that world, and frequently was excused as being necessary to reduce the constant stress in our day and night lives. If certain actions were disrespectful to women, so be it. The institution and the culture it engendered simply did not take women or their feelings into account. There was no need to. As very special beings, surgeons were protected—and the institution paid the bills. Had I voiced any objection, I would have derailed my career in surgery almost as rapidly as I would have by becoming pregnant. What else was there to do but join in— and have a good time?

On the work front, some faculty surgeons enjoyed testing me by giving me difficult cases, such as a gallbladder or splenectomy, as opposed to hernias or hemorrhoidectomies, which are the cases usually done by those with the least experience. This turned out to be an advantage: by the time I finished two years of general surgery, I had done more difficult cases than had my male resident peers and the operative experience has served me well. Mostly, however, I do not think I was taken seriously by the surgeons who taught me, and many treated me like "a cute little piece of fluff," more suitable for romance than for blood and guts. I was often asked, without a trace of subtlety, when I planned to start a family. I had the distinct impression that few thought board certification as a surgeon lay in my future. At the end of a six-month general surgery rotation at the VA, the Chief of Surgery, a professor, told me I was a good surgeon, but way too aggressive for his tastes. My future would be easier for everyone, including me, he said, if I could develop restraint and a degree of feminine shyness. It was impossible to think his advice was in my best interest. My successful compatriots were anything but shy. I saw a pushy assertiveness as being the best way to get ahead. Yet I could ignore being patronized and accept it with grace because I believed if I developed good talent as a surgeon, that alone would be sufficient to conquer old ingrained prejudices. I was not about to let others limit my dreams, and thus copied the behavior I thought would allow me to realize them.

Phil's life probably would have been easier had I stuck with my original intent of becoming a plastic surgeon. Unfortunately, when I rotated on to plastic surgery for the required month during my internship, I had found the subject boring—the surgery itself is great fun, but the basic subject matter was not intellectually demanding enough for my taste. There was an ugly scar on an arm, the breasts were too small, or the nose was too big. Taking care of burn patients in that era was a truly hideous experience. Even today I can smell the silver nitrate solution, used to clean the burn, mingling with the scent of scorched, dying flesh, the silver paradoxically turning everything it touched black, except for the yellow-red depths of the wound itself. After morning rounds with the attending plastic surgeon professor, it fell to the intern to return for a daily torture session of cutting dead tissue from the burn, the anguished cries of pain never sufficiently dulled by Demerol or morphine.

Unexpectedly, during my month as the neurosurgical intern, I found neurosurgery to be the most exciting discipline I had ever encountered. It had everything. In the pre-CT, pre-MRI scan era, a neurosurgeon had to be an exacting diagnostician, asking where the nervous system was hurt; why or what was causing the incapacity; and what, if anything, could be done to reverse the damage. Unlike neurologists, who spend as much or more time intellectualizing about neurologic dysfunction as they do attempting to treat it, neurosurgeons have the technical ability to reverse many devastating neurologic deficits with surgery. A paralyzed patient walks, a mute stroke patient talks, a tumor patient borrows extra time. I knew then this was what I wanted to do with my life.

But in the 1960s almost no surgical programs were taking any women into their ranks, let alone into neurosurgery. There were no prohibitive written policies in place—women were just not expected to have any interest in surgery, and certainly did not belong there. Plastic surgery had been a gentle compromise for those who otherwise would have unilaterally denied my desire to wield a scalpel. No one thought to tell me I could not be a neurosurgeon—the very idea had never been considered. Had I sought Phil's advice ahead of time, which I deliberately did not do, I think he would have employed powerful persuasive arguments against the switch I made.

The chair of neurosurgery, Dr. John (Jake) Hanbery, walked with a pronounced limp on a leg foreshortened by a childhood bout of osteomyelitis, and had a markedly receding chin line that kept his face from being handsome. A pipe was his constant playmate, amusing hands and mouth, and molecules of pipe tobacco were buried layers deep in every inch of his skin. The smell of pipe smoke had defined "neurosurgeon" for the rest of the hospital ever since 1959. Hanbery hid excessive shyness behind a gruff exterior, and socially was rarely at ease. I found him very intimidating, as did most others. But he was the only one who could approve a change in my residency program from plastic surgery to neurosurgery. I did realize my request would be unexpected, unwelcome, and even laughable.

No one told me not to bother Dr. Hanbery at noontime, although, in retrospect, all except me seemed to know what went on in his office during that sacred hour. I had chosen midday deliberately, and was naively unfazed when I found the door to his office shut. After all, some read or sleep in their offices, in addition to eating, during the programmed quiet of lunchtime. My intrusive knock seemed very loud in the silence. In response to it, I heard unexpected muffled voices. After a few seconds, Hanbery came to the door and opened it a head width. "Yeah?" he asked, while tying the drawstring of a pair of scrub pants around his waist, his usually neatly combed, thinning dark hair unruly and rumpled. My thoughts started racing: "My God, what've I gotten into?" I caught a glimpse—but it was enough—of his secretary on the sofa behind him, and lowered my eyes.

Blushing with embarrassment for both of us, I blurted out, "I want to go into neurosurgery, can I have a place in your program?"

"Oh sure—yeah, sure," he answered, and slammed the door shut. To his credit, Professor Hanbery honored his promise and gave me the one open position as the newest of seven residents in his neurosurgical training program.

That evening I told Phil I had changed residency programs. Even though I waited until he had enjoyed his first glass of wine, he was aghast. "Why do you have to pick the goddamnedest most difficult thing you can think of?" he inquired, without a great deal of gentility. But it was what I really wanted to do and he was smart enough to know it.

My joining the neurosurgery residency program in 1966 was viewed with marked alarm by the residents already in the program. Prior to making the switch I had not considered the personalities of those who were in training or the fact that I would have to work closely with a number of them. Years later I learned there had been a hastily convened dinner meeting where they, along with three neurosurgeons who had graduated from the program and who were in private practice in the local area, discussed my intrusion into their all-white-male domain. It had been more a "My God, what's the world come to?" session than a meeting to plan strategy for righting the perceived wrong. All knew Jake Hanbery was a man of his word, and if he had promised a place to me, the place was mine. However, his judgment, as well as his sanity, was open to question.

Professor Hanbery was a dominant figure in our medical world, both feared and revered by those who trained under him. He was a gifted neurosurgeon and a marvelous teacher of both surgical technique and patient assessment. But his work bias was old-fashioned and dictatorial. On the wards and in the operating room he always adhered to a rigid pecking order, addressing all remarks exclusively to his chief resident, who, in turn, would direct the work of the junior resident and intern. During my years as a junior resident, I worked with a number of trainees, including two very different chief residents.

Nothing I did was ever good enough for the first chief resident. Doug Pontis was an unmarried workaholic with a twenty-four-hour-per-day total devotion to neurosurgery, interrupted only by Mass on Sunday mornings. He expected the same time commitment from me, even though, to him, I had no legitimate place in surgery—instead, I was his slave, and his was the only right way. I would find him at 3 a.m. on the ward writing an addendum to one of my patient assessments, adding a picayune item I had neglected or even chosen to omit. Occasionally, we would disagree over the correct diagnosis. If I, rather than he, proved correct, three days of sullen silence would follow. I was allowed to do almost no surgical cases, and spent a year of negative professional growth wondering what I was doing in neurosurgery. Fortunately, once he finished his year as chief resident, Doug left the academic world to enter private practice, and thus was out of my life. Unfortunately, his firmly fixed ideas about the proper role in life for a woman were shared by many male surgeons, including fellow resident Gerry Silverberg, whom I had initially encountered a year or so before while I was a medical student.

I had come across Gerry while he was doing a required year of general surgery before starting his neurosurgery training. At that time he was a constant source of conversation in the emergency room. ER doctors and other surgeons gossiped over their cups of coffee about the humorous, and sometimes outrageous, behavior of this first-year surgical resident. Once I heard about him, I naturally looked for him and then could not help but watch him. I was fascinated by his unusual behavior, by the way he played the critical fool, demanding the center of attention, always noticeable, dominant, and up-front. He was very self-assured, laughed frequently and easily, and was very generous with sarcastic comments. Even as a lowly first-year resident he carried an aura of lofty self-importance—he was, after all, in training to become a neurosurgeon, and did not hesitate to inform anyone who would listen about his ambitious plans for a brilliant career as one of the country's best.

As fellow neurosurgical residents we now had frequent contact, although Gerry and I never served on a clinical service together. Because he had graduated from Stanford two years ahead of me, we spent a number of overlapping years as residents, and subsequently have served many years as fellow faculty members. As part of his basic persona Gerry loved to tease and test me, always for an audience. He would invite me to go to bed with him, thrust his pelvis forward, look down at and directly ask his genitals if they would like that, then laugh, and wait for a response from me. The invitations were never serious or taken seriously, and were never extended in private. At times his antics were so incredible they made me and others laugh—standing there giggling while offering me a gift of the mound showing beneath his tightly fitted scrub greens. Frequently, over the years, usually out of earshot of the patient, I have heard the penis proffered as the miraculous cure for many disorders suffered by women, especially those afflicting young, attractive ones. Numerous times in informal groups on rounds or in the clinic area, Gerry would amuse us by bragging about his sexual conquests, or would whine that his workload had been so heavy he had been forced to be true blue to his wife.

In marked contrast to Doug's and Gerry's attitude, Jason Runyon, the second chief resident I worked with, opened the world of neurosurgery for me, not as an abstraction, which it had been prior to then, but as reality. He also let me know that I had a legitimate place in that world if I was willing to work for it. Once we were doing a difficult case at the VA (Dr. Hanbery was not in the operating room, trusting Jason to call him if he needed help) and Jason was struggling to position an operating microscope optimally. With the impatience of youth I suggested he forget the bloody scope and do the case without it. Instead of anger at my totally improper outburst, with infinite patience Jason turned to me and said, "You and I are going to do this case correctly, using whatever it takes to make things as safe as possible for this patient." My face flushed a deep red behind my surgical mask and I shut up—I had been chastised, as was perfectly appropriate. But, at the same time, Jason had included me as a fellow neurosurgeon.

Phil and Jason became good friends. They shared athletic interests, and each had a wife with a strong sense of herself. Although Phil was aware I sometimes felt diminished and belittled by Gerry and his sexist behavior, on social occasions he and others, including Jason, found Gerry quite charming. He had a good sense of humor, was entertaining, a passable dancer, and could tell a good story. However, Phil would occasionally take issue with some of Gerry's derogatory comments, such as questioning how anyone could expect much from a mere woman. He would offer to intervene on my behalf and put Gerry in his place. More than once I asked Phil to "cool it," because, especially in the early years of my residency, when I felt like such a freak, an outburst from him would have meant goodbye to neurosurgery for me. A vocal, dissatisfied spouse, male or female, could catalyze dismissal of a resident from his or her training program. Over the years, two residents left our program after their wives made late-night phone calls to Dr. Hanbery at his home, hysterically yelling and screaming about how hard their husbands were having to work. Gradually Phil learned medical spouses were "onstage" too, and they were expected to suffer the loss of their mates to the incessant demands of the hospital in martyred silence. An additional burden for spouses was to pretend enthusiasm for an abusive schedule of physician training that encompassed severe sleep deprivation and no consistent time off for regathering one's soul. For my (our) sake, Phil kept quiet.

In my fourth year of residency Phil abruptly terminated his employment, having decided he did not enjoy punching someone else's time clock. I was totally panicked. I was not making enough money as a resident physician to support the two of us, but "not to worry," Phil said. He founded his own financial advising and consulting company, carefully choosing clients with both money and interesting financial and investment problems. His low-key, half-vocational, half-avocational business thrived, finding a home at home, and in addition to "making money with money," he developed expertise as a consummate househusband. He did all the grocery shopping and prepared most of our meals. Friends thought his life very weird, and more than one told him he was being cheated with regard to his marriage contract. Some were just plain envious—Phil now had complete control over his daily time clock. But his lifestyle was not seen as legitimate, and certainly not very manly. However, from the time Phil deserted his own conventional career, *my* career became *our* career, and he has been an active participant in my professional development since. He keeps me tethered to the real world, and is quick to delineate, then castigate, the inconsistencies, abuses, and outright fantasies and flaws that characterize the very bizarre world of academic medicine.

Distance running had become a social, as well as a psychological and physical outlet for us. With a group of friends we entered the annual Bay-to-Breakers footrace across San Francisco in 1971, the first year women were officially allowed to participate. I had gone to the city to run the 7.8-mile race for fun, and had not really thought about the competition. Unexpectedly, I was the first woman to cross the finish line, and, over the years, winning this race has been my "main claim to fame." As I struggled to catch my breath, the waiting press had only two questions for me: "Are you married?" and "Where do you live?" The newspaper article the following day informed its readership that a "Palo Alto housewife" had won the women's race, despite the fact that I was an M.D. halfway through an eight-year neurosurgical training program. How could they know that one of Phil's favorite comments, said with a smile to guests at our home, was, "In this house, a doctor cleans the toilets!"

In 1973, Dr. Hanbery asked Gerry Silverberg to join him on the faculty to help with a rapidly increasing clinical load. It was an invitation Gerry had expected ever since his internship years before. During my year as chief resident, he and Hanbery were my teachers, and I learned a great deal from him. Gerry had developed into a savvy technical neurosurgeon. He did difficult cases, his patients did well, and he pioneered new operative techniques. But he was never able to develop a noteworthy research program—in fairness, he was encumbered with heavy clinical responsibilities and was not offered protected research time. The lack of a research component hurt him at promotion hurdles. He owed, in every sense of the word, his academic career to Dr. Hanbery. He was awarded tenure and kept on the faculty only because Dr. Hanbery threatened to resign if Gerry was not promoted. Dr. Hanbery told the dean he would establish a competing practice across the street in partnership with Gerry. Neurosurgery brought in considerable money, a percentage of which accrued to the dean in the form of an internal tax. The threat of relative poverty forced the dean to capitulate.

I too owed my career to Professor Hanbery. For years he suffered outwardly good-natured but serious ribbing from colleagues for having taken a woman into his program. Not only did he train me but in 1975 he unexpectedly asked me to join the faculty. He and Gerry had grown tired of covering both Stanford and the VA on a daily basis, and decided to rid themselves of the latter inconvenience by adding a third faculty member. When the invitation was offered I had been exploring private practice opportunities and had not previously seriously considered an academic career. In addition to being named assistant professor at Stanford University, I was also asked to take over as chief of the Section of Neurosurgery at the fully affiliated VA hospital in Palo Alto, with responsibility for directing its program of residency training. I divided my time between the two facilities. I operated and ran a clinic at both places, but maintained my main office and established a research enterprise at the VA.

Dr. Hanbery had always been an aloof and not very approachable person. Initially I believe he was ambivalent about whether I would, or even should, succeed in academics—I had been hired primarily to make his and Gerry's lives easier. While grudgingly supportive in the early years, he never provided me with information about academic process, never held a performance review with me, nor did he provide start-up money for my research program. In order to qualify for tenure, a nationally recognized research effort was essential, but I was left either to make it or not on my own at the VA. Were one to confront Dr. Hanbery about this apparent lack of formal performance evaluation and constructive help, he would have answered, "I'll let her know if she does something wrong." It was the way he functioned in his academic world.

I had become a comfortable fixture at the medical school during my long, eight-year residency. Once my faculty appointment was secure (I was the first and only female in any of the surgical disciplines), the Department of Surgery elected me to represent it as a member of the Medical Faculty Senate. Since I had not yet proven myself as a faculty member, I thought my fellow surgeons were telling the rest of the medical school, "Hey, we can be avant-garde and are more than willing to join this newfangled, changing world." I also felt there was an element of "Look what we've got—isn't she cute?" in their behavior. At the first meeting of the Senate, I was, to my great surprise, elected its chair. Never before had the chair been a nontenured member of the faculty, let alone a woman. The dean's office insisted that memos about Senate business be addressed to me as "chairman," despite my clearly articulated preference for "chair." With a bit of rudimentary feminism, I believed then, and certainly do today, that language is a profound indicator of value.

As chair I became a voting member of the dean's Executive Committee (composed of all the department chairs) and had access to all its confidential information, including promotion and appointment data about other faculty members. I learned more about the requirements for tenure at Stanford Medical School by reviewing promotion papers than from any other source. Fortunately for me, the information supplanted the need to find a personal mentor or to bother Dr. Hanbery. I had no role models—there simply were no academic women around in my surgical world, and I did not search beyond it. However, I rapidly learned others considered me to be a role model for them, even though, in the early years, I had grave doubts about my own survival as an academician. Tenure was, and is, very difficult to earn at Stanford University.

Shortly after I joined the faculty, the Dean of Students asked me to meet with a female medical student who had encountered some interpersonal problems on her surgical clerkship. She was being subjected to what I had come to recognize as the usual verbal diatribe from Stanford's male surgeons: "Dollface, you should be home raising beautiful children," and "Why would anyone with your looks want to be here doing this messy work?" While she scrubbed her hands and arms at the sink, the faculty surgeon, who waited to wash his hands until his surgical skill was needed in the case, would give her an uninvited neck massage and whisper in her ear, "Wish I could be doing this with you somewhere else." The Dean of Students had no intention of changing the behavior of the surgeons; that was the way they were. I was to counsel her so *she* could adapt to the operating room—a rite of passage for every female medical student. I remember being quite surprised by how offended she had been. After all, the operating room nurses tolerated worse abuses; her breasts were not being fondled, her crotch was not being grabbed, she had not been propositioned. Her complaints were about behavior I experienced every day, and I was of no help to her, giving her the standard litany of "toughen up or you're not going to make it." She left my office close to tears—I had been anything but the ally she expected, and she was profoundly disappointed. Changing the surgeon's world was not part of my agenda. So I defended it. How could a lowly, know-nothing medical student know enough to criticize it? I did believe that as numbers of women increased in a particular arena, discrimination and sexism would decrease. So with time, inevitably the surgical culture would also change, although I never gave any thought as to how rapidly, or even when. Since I saw no evidence of imminent change, I decided it was better to put up with it and shut up.

Every Thursday at noon the entire surgical faculty gathered for lunch, and, until I joined them in 1975, the meetings were a loud vocal stag party. Faculty surgeons who were not otherwise occupied in the operating room would converge for free food and raucous humor, to share the latest dirty jokes, and to hear an update about the state of the surgical department and the school. Politically these were important meetings to attend. One acquired information and solidified and authenticated one's membership as "surgeon." I desperately wanted to belong, and never tried to diminish my colleagues' "fun." The meetings were, at times, downright disgusting and the "humor" frequently was at my expense.

The group would sit around a large, long table, and one of the surgeons would play a favorite game if he happened to take the seat next to me. He would place a caressing hand on my knee and begin moving it up my thigh. The action was overt—everyone in the room knew what was happening. I would grab his offensive fingers and place his hand, with a loud thump, back on the table where it belonged, and where everyone could see it. At the same time the caresser would be told to "keep your goddamn hand to yourself." Everyone, including me, laughed. After all, none of this was serious, he meant no real harm. The group delighted in having this game played repeatedly and I could not always control who sat on either side of me.

During the luncheons, the surgeons spent considerable time insulting each other over sexual prowess, or, more often, its apparent lack, egging each other on to ever more outlandish, ribald comments. Urologists in the group were pressured, humorously, to divulge information about their colleagues' ability in bed, or whether or not they could still "get it up." These noontime sessions did expand my entertainment repertoire with some of the funniest dirty jokes I have ever heard.

I was well prepared for the inevitable skirmish, which, on occasion, I won. Once a noted surgeon and I were each building a sandwich and I looked at his, then back at mine, and said, innocently, making idle conversation, "Mine looks better than yours." Without a moment's hesitation, he answered, "And I'll bet it's longer and stiffer too." I flipped him the finger, much to his and the crowd's delight. On another occasion, as I entered the room for lunch, a male colleague yelled out, "I can see the shape of your breasts and nipples even through that white coat!" All eyes turned to appraise my fully, and nonprovocatively, clothed body. My face turned red, and an appropriate, incisively belittling reply, for a moment, failed me. Then I answered, "And I noticed yours is hanging on the left today, sir!"

For the most part I enjoyed these noon meetings, finding psychic survival to be a challenging, toughening experience. I realized only much later, rather than being considered a surgeon, I was instead seen as an embarrassed, compromised sex object—but one that could usually hold her own.

In general, surgeons are gregarious, friendly individuals when they are with each other. While at work, most would rather be in an operating room than in any other place, such as in the clinic or emergency room, where they have to deal face to face with patients. The environment in an operating room is rigidly controlled, and every participant has well-defined duties. The surgeon is "king," the patient is asleep, the anesthesiologist is viewed as a lesser professional, and the nursing staff is obsequiously subservient. It is a culture that breeds arrogance, rigidity, and an inflated sense of self-worth. It is small wonder that many surgeons do not develop an engaging "bedside manner," and see patients as objects rather than as people with feelings, pain, desires, and fear. Objects are far easier to control when they are bereft of emotionality. A surgeon's value is in his surgical skill, not in having to be nice to people. Thus surgeons are most comfortable with their fellow "kings," because they have a commonality of experience in having perfect, delicious control over what they do on a daily basis.

During residency, and later as faculty, I had known about and witnessed episodes of blatant discrimination and harassment of women by surgeons. Some of the outwardly nicest, seemingly kindest men become total maniacs in an operating room, where they have absolute power to act out almost any way they desire. Operating room nurses are especially vulnerable to the whims of a surgeon. Seductiveness is combined and interspersed with temper tantrums, instrument throwing, abusive name calling, and irrational requests. Some treat their nursing staff like little dogs, often reducing them to whimpering, cowering creatures whose large, timid eyes fill and overflow with tears and whose tails remain firmly tucked between their legs. When scrubbed for a case a nurse cannot use her hands to fight unwelcome advances unless she is willing to break a sterile field and potentially endanger an unconscious patient. It is not a democratic society. A nurse and her actions are subject to unilateral criticism from a surgeon after a case is finished, followed by a stinging reprimand from a nursing supervisor—anything to keep the almighty surgeon happy.

Thus, most OR nurses I saw kept quiet and endured the abuse without complaining. It made life much easier. I too swallowed hard and accepted the episodes I witnessed as being part of that peculiar environment.

Woman-as-surgeon has never been a part of this surgeon tableau. The women surgeons I know, for the most part, have avoided developing the bad interpersonal traits exhibited by some of their male colleagues, and most have an engaging touch with patients. Many male surgeons seem uncertain about how they should treat or communicate with a female surgeon and where she really fits. She is not subject to the same control he has over nurses, but she also is not equivalent to him or to his male surgical colleagues. Not uncommonly, "humorous" flirting is used, more or less unconsciously, to establish her inferior status in his own mind (this is also uniformly true when he deals with nurses). Many surgeons have no understanding of why they have a compulsive need to flirt.

During residency I had been consumed by the job and need for sleep, in that order. The Vietnam War and the student activism it spawned had come and gone without causing any blip in my cloistered, focused life. Phil had been happy when I accepted Dr. Hanbery's offer of employment, but mistakenly believed that a faculty position would provide more free time for both of us. It did not. I no longer had to do all the routine "scut" details of patient care twenty-four hours a day, leaving those chores to the interns and residents. But life was now occupied with equally time-consuming patient assessment, operative decisions, surgeries, and total responsibility for many patients' lives, along with a growing research enterprise studying the immunology of brain tumors, where laboratory animals had to be observed 365 days a year. Intrusions from my beeper and nighttime phone calls remained an integral part of my life.

Every academic is also expected to teach. While I give the

occasional standard-format lecture to preclinical students, my teaching is predominantly tutorial, and almost exclusively at the resident level. Until 1988 all the residents in our program were white and male. That year, to fill a sudden vacancy, a female medical student who had matched in neurology but who had expressed a strong interest in transferring to neurosurgery was added to our program. Thus, for the majority of years of my academic career, the residents I trained were men with a variable degree of willingness to follow directions from me—or from the other faculty. Only once, early in my career, have I ever ordered a resident to leave the OR—he was totally uncooperative, insisted he could do the case without assistance or direction from me, and was, I thought, endangering the patient. He was asked to leave our training program shortly thereafter—I was not alone in having problems with him. Resident behavior is somewhat controlled by fear generated from hierarchical order. All faculty, regardless of gender, possess the power to make or break a resident.

During my residency I had spent minimal time contemplating any role as a teacher in a future professional setting, but I rapidly learned to adapt and adjust to each new resident, melding my personality peculiarities with theirs. Some residents need to develop increased aggressiveness; others, more commonly, need to be held back. One acquires an instinct about how much tether to give each resident, when to back off, and when to apply a sharp jerk to the chain. The patient's welfare is always the number one priority, and an operating team that works well together and understands each other achieves the best results.

One of the first cases I did as a faculty member was on a twenty-eight-year-old man who had suffered from a seizure disorder since childhood. He had been referred to me when a CT scan (Stanford had acquired its first clinical scanner in 1974, a year before I finished my residency) revealed that his epilepsy was caused by a tangled knot of abnormal arteries and veins in his brain, called an arteriovenous malformation (AVM). Total excision of these lesions usually makes seizures easier to control with medication and eliminates the threat of a future brain hemorrhage. While removing the abnormality the resident working with me and I alternated positions between being operating surgeon and assistant, and a number of times I admonished him that he was in danger of losing his left one (testicle) if he did not stay closer to the AVM in line with my verbal directions. The hypothetical threat was one I used frequently and almost unconsciously—yes, I am burdened with my own set of faults. Surgery went quite smoothly, but was exacting and intricate and took eight hours to perform. Postoperatively, the patient looked terrific. Before going home that evening around 9 p.m., I dropped in for a last-minute check on his condition. He was talking to me about his father when he abruptly stopped in mid-sentence, and rapidly became deeply unconscious. The resident and I rushed him back to the operating room and removed a blood clot that had formed in the resection bed in his brain. We finished at 1 a.m. When he awoke, his left side was paralyzed. I was devastated—things had gone so well during the first surgery, and he should have been completely normal. What had gone wrong? Had we not controlled the bleeding carefully enough at the end of the case? Had we left part of the AVM behind, allowing its fragile vessel walls to break and bleed? While the resident had been somewhat overconfident about his skills during surgery, he was very uncomfortable managing this case that had gone sour. So the remainder of that truncated night's sleep was interrupted by numerous phone calls for decisions about controlling the patient's blood pressure, his breathing, his blood count and neurologic status. At 7:30 the next morning, I started the first of three cases which had previously been scheduled for that day. The patient with the AVM remained completely paralyzed for an agonizing three days, then had gradual return of some function and was able to ambulate awkwardly, but without assistance, when he left the hospital.

During my career, both men and women have served as surgical
interns, but, when they rotate on to our service for their month
of neurosurgery, they are primarily responsible for the care of
patients on the wards and spend only minimal time in the operating room. The occasional medical student (both genders, but
more men than women) will serve an elective clerkship on neurosurgery, gaining some operative experience, but their time with
us is short, and they are so intimidated by the whole scene they
will do whatever is asked of them without asking questions. Even
with this skewed database, I find, in general, that women are less
aggressive as surgeons (certainly at the beginning of their careers)
and far more willing to ask for help and follow directions than
are men.

I was able to establish control over work activities at the VA and
Stanford, but after joining the faculty I rapidly learned how much
of an unwelcome novelty I would be to the "old guard" of my
peer group of academic neurosurgeons away from Stanford. After
being on the faculty for a year, I submitted a paper from my
fledgling research program for presentation at a meeting of the
American Association of Neurological Surgeons (AANS), one of
our two national organizations. Amazingly, it was accepted for
one of the prestigious plenary sessions. I was absolutely thrilled,
and scared to death.

I find national meetings miserable affairs, held in a variety of
nameless cities, at sterile, overpriced hotels. Scientific presentations are given in huge ballrooms filled with stale, cold, air-
conditioned air to an audience haphazardly distributed in row
upon row of uncomfortable folding chairs. Behavior of neurosurgeons at these gatherings resembles that of a bunch of stallions
in heat, as the ritual to establish a new, current rank order is
repeated year after year. Neurosurgeons have huge egos. Friends

become two-faced strangers as they self-promote, backstab, and vie with each other for recognition. In general, women have not learned how to advertise themselves or their accomplishments in this way, and, as such, are ill equipped to play this game. The scarce female neurosurgeon is left without an assigned ranking, understandably and almost inexorably relegating her to the periphery of the profession.

At that first meeting I was so alone, even though surrounded by suits. I knew almost no one, and had no one to make introductions for me, as Dr. Hanbery had chosen to skip the meeting. After I presented my paper, Dr. Roget, an eminent neurosurgeon whom I knew by reputation only, hailed me and asked me to discuss my research program with him. I was ecstatic. He asked me to sit because he said he could not talk to women when they were standing. I obediently sat down. He told me he thought it was marvelous that the AANS program committee had decided to include an immunologist on the program. He continued by saying that neurosurgeons really are pretty uninformed about immunology, and do not know it can be used to look at and maybe even treat some diseases of the nervous system.

"I'm sorry, Dr. Roget," I interrupted with some pride. "I'm not an immunologist. I'm a neurosurgeon on the faculty at Stanford Medical School." He jerked back in his chair as if I had slapped his face, peered imperiously at me over half-frame spectacles, and without another word stood up and rapidly walked away to join three of his male colleagues. After a moment of disbelief, I asked myself what in hell I was doing in this strange world.

I experienced a sudden wave of uncertainty about my future, along with profound loneliness. Dr. Roget's behavior told me the image just did not compute for him. It was my first conscious realization that role stereotyping is the most powerful force affecting the career of a woman surgeon. No matter how good you are, if you do not look the part the automatic assumption is you cannot play the part. Interestingly, surgical peers have more difficulty dispelling this stereotyped image and thinking than do patients. In my experience as a surgeon, patients have accepted me almost without question, primarily because of their perception that I had to be "better than the boys" to have made it.

Dr. Roget had been able to visualize me in the role of a female research immunologist, but the thought of my opening someone's head to mess around with a brain just was not part of his definition of "woman's work." That I, a woman, could develop and present a scientific paper as a neurosurgeon was unfathomable to him.

A pivotal component of an academic career revolves around a research laboratory, research funding, research results, and publications, especially those in highly prestigious journals. In truth, probably no more than a few dozen other scientists, working in the same field, have ever read any of the publications generated by my laboratory, yet academic success, especially in medicine, is welded to an investigative enterprise which produces published papers—and continued grant support. Once my laboratory was established, I published regularly, and for sixteen years managed to obtain uninterrupted monetary support from competitive grants.

With my gender-neutral first name, for years I was referred to as "he" in grant critiques from funding agencies. My first name would be spelled correctly on the front sheet, but the summary would read, "Dr. Conley has been quite productive, and his present proposal is well written and he provides good experimental detail. He is well trained and has a good bibliography." I often wonder how much research funding I received was for being a good research scientist as opposed to being a good *male* research scientist. Maybe I should thank the name my parents gave me for my research career. Maybe I could have done even better had I not relinquished my maiden name, in order to capitalize on my father's reputation with a last name recognized by the National Academy of Sciences. Perhaps I should have written a polite, or even indignant, letter to the granting agency, stating, "For your records, I am a 'she,' not a 'he.' " But I feared such action might have insulted those who controlled my academic future, resulting in a lower score on my next grant application, followed by a decrease or cutoff of funding. So I kept my mouth shut, laughed, and felt sorry for women named Susie or Mary Ann. After all, I had learned how to play this game and thought I was thriving.

By the time of my tenure review in 1982, Phil and I had decided, without any formal discussion about the pros and cons, that we would not have children. Having children never seemed to fit into our lives—I was always a student, an intern, a resident, or a faculty person, driven to succeed. So instead of having our own, Phil and I "adopted" grown children, students at Stanford, usually student athletes. For many years we nurtured our "kids" psychologically, and, on occasion, financially, and take great pride in their subsequent achievements as business, legal, and medical professionals. Our daily surrogate "children" have been a succession of both dogs and cats—dearly beloved little creatures who share their uncompromised love and devotion and liberally enrich our lives.

An untraditional family life was one of the trade-offs we informally accepted with each other so I could build an academic career, without need to compromise on the standard amount of time required for a decision about tenure. I wanted an unbroken path of credentials and accomplishments, without excuses or absences, a record that would read as having been played entirely by the prevailing (masculine) rules: an academician not burdened by child care responsibilities and, additionally, having a supportive spouse—at home. The few married women academics I saw at Stanford were expected to have children, and when they did, they gracefully stepped off their committed career paths to be mothers for whatever time it took. The problem was that, once off, they never got back on. They spent their many productive academic years as Senior Research Associates rather than as full professors. At the time of my tenure review I had not produced a child, so I had to be viewed as someone who ostensibly was there for the long haul, someone who was competitive along with the rest of them, someone for whom no given set of rules really applied. Interestingly, for the career woman, both childbearing and childlessness are regarded negatively. However, it would have been far less threatening for many, I believe, had I chosen motherhood, and only secondarily pursued a more leisurely nonacademic career in neurosurgery.

I was awarded tenure in 1982, almost on time, but not without some personal turmoil. A tenure review is a very emotional experience for any candidate—it determines if one has an academic future. I knew the review had been started, but was not informed of milestones along the way—an experience that was not unique to me. One of my earliest childhood memories is of when my father had been awarded tenure years before. At that time my folks threw a happy party with friends packed into the formal living room (where children were not usually allowed) and spilling out onto the large covered porch (which was our play yard on rainy days). I vividly remember the adult mess made with bottles of champagne, the sound and sight of popping corks, the white head of frothy wine spilling over the thick glass mouth to form a bubbling cascade down the sides of the bottle. Significantly, no one yelled at all the funny people for spilling on the rug when the bubbles were not captured quite quickly enough. I had enjoyed just being there, in that special room, among the pant legs and skirt hems of my child world, looking up at friendly, warm faces, accepting sips of champagne and rewarding those who shared with increasingly tipsy little-girl giggles.

In 1982 I had hoped to relive my memory and celebrate a positive tenure decision in June, but heard nothing as the month came and went. As my worry and concern increased, I asked my father to make some discreet inquiries—fortunately he was there when I needed him and few in our university community knew we were related. It turns out the professor of medicine who was chair of my tenure committee had gone on vacation without convening his group beforehand. I was not informed of this delay, which had nothing whatever to do with my suitability for a tenured appointment. A favorable decision was reached in early September, but after the uncertainty and mental distress, and in marked contrast to my father's happiness at the time of his tenure award, Phil and I felt there was no need to waste even a single bottle of champagne over mine.

Shortly after the tenure decision, one of my surgical professor friends, eight years older than I, one day unexpectedly asked me, "Fran, why isn't what you have good enough?" I do not believe he would have asked a male academic the same question. Men are expected to be competitive, to advance their careers as rapidly and as far as possible. Initially I considered my friend's comment a compliment—it implied I had done far more than he ever thought I would, especially given the environment I had chosen to work in. After mulling it over, however, I grasped his hidden meaning. I had not heard it, because I did not want to believe it. He was telling me I had come far enough, thank you, and should stop before I became any more of a competitive threat—after all, now that I had tenure my academic position was secure, guaranteed for life, and there was no need to accomplish more. I would be happier, the school would be happier, the academic world would be happier, were I to fade contentedly into the woodwork and live out my academic career as a well-behaved, good little girl. The rules governing my work should have been gender-neutral—I had as much right to the work and the rewards as anyone else. But more than once over the years I had been told in all seriousness that I did not need to be paid as much because I was married. Of course, the doctors who told me so were also married and occasionally their wives even worked. I thought they were kidding. I was putting in just as many hours as everyone else, and had always pulled my fair share of night and weekend calls. I deciphered their true message only much later. They considered my getting rousted out of bed at 3 a.m. to care for a patient to be not worth as much as similar care provided by one of my male neurosurgical colleagues. I now know the medical system has always assigned increased value to work done by men.

In 1984, Dr. David Korn, professor and chair of the Department of Pathology, was appointed dean of the School of Medicine. Faculty had been divided over the selection. The final choice between a clinician and a basic scientist was driven more by who could attract the most research money than by personality or competence in managing people. The humanistic component that is the real force behind any first-rate medical school, and that had been found in former occupants of the dean's office, was forgotten in the excitement generated by an era of proliferating biomedical research. For the first years of Dr. Korn's deanship, the medical school built its enviable reputation as a world-renowned research institution, and was able to attract the most highly regarded young medical research scholars and scientists. Money flowed, buildings were constructed, institutes and corporations fought among themselves for the privilege of a resource partnership with Stanford University's prestigious medical school. It was a glorious, golden era, a time when Dean Korn made a flippant remark to me at a reception after he had enjoyed a couple of glasses of wine to the effect that wouldn't this be a wonderful place if we didn't have to worry about students and clinical faculty?

I took a year of sabbatical leave in 1985–86. The practice of medicine was changing with the advent of managed care. I wanted to understand the future and be prepared for it. In a move I thought would build career strength, and with Phil's enthusiastic support, I went to Stanford's business school for the year to learn skills that would enhance my ability to make decisions about the future of medicine, especially were I to end up in an administrative position. More and more doctors were finding value in having some business education. Just prior to my starting, Dean Korn had told me humorously that I should take over his job as dean for a year and that *he* should be the one going to business school.

In my Sloan program, a one year Master's degree in Management Science, I learned that survival in business meant understanding and keeping pace with all aspects of the external world, the ability to make decisions based on incomplete information, a willingness to take risks, and the availability of accurate cost-benefit analyses. Dynamic change was rewarded; complacency led to failure. I studied finance, cost accounting, strategic planning, organizational behavior, and how to analyze power. Professor Jeffrey Pfeffer taught the class on power. The taboo subject was mesmerizing. We learned to analyze organizations through the way management used and recognized power. Who has it? How did they get it? How is it identified or validated within the organization? Is it shared, and, if so, how, with whom, and why? How is it used? And, finally, how is it lost? Because I recognized the tenets Professor Pfeffer taught were applicable to a far wider arena than business, I invited him to explore power dynamics in the VA operating rooms the summer after I received my degree. My particular interest was to determine if male and female surgeons used dissimilar forms of "power" in their surgical domains. I was convinced my style in the operating room was quite different from that of my male neurosurgical colleagues.

Jeff rapidly became a fixture in the surgical suite, someone who was there but could be ignored, the consummate observant psychologist. He found watching surgery boring, but was fascinated by hierarchical interplay in the operating room. He rarely observed me (I was the only woman neurosurgeon, so comparisons were impossible) but chose instead to spend most of his time with general surgeons at the VA, where women were represented both as faculty and as residents. To no one's real surprise, Jeff found there were definite stereotypical gender differences. Male surgeons were top-down, dictatorial managers, "captains of the ship," who frequently used anger to obtain obedience from their nursing staff. Women surgeons, almost uniformly, used a consensual management style. The staff worked together as a team to complete a task (the operation). Anger was rare; instead, a bantering type of humor prevailed. Significantly, both management styles yielded equivalent end results—a well-performed operation and a satisfied patient.

Anger is a powerful management tool and Jeff was intrigued by its differential use by male and female surgeons. He asked me what I did if I was genuinely angry. My answer: "If I'm angry, really, really angry, I let it explode—then it's very effective, because I use anger so very sparingly the rest of the time." Most of the time I feel prohibited from using anger, and often internalize exasperation rather than vent my displeasure. Another pointed observation Jeff made was, "My God, you people touch each other a lot, and I'm not talking about when you're with patients. You touch one another at times and in ways that would be totally unacceptable in any other occupational environment I can think of."

The year at the business school away from neurosurgery (although not from my laboratory, which maintained a high level of productivity) provided a marvelous time of intellectual growth for me. It was such fun to learn a new language, new approaches, to think and write creatively again. During the year I learned Gerry had informed mutual friends at national meetings of neurosurgeons that I was abandoning neurosurgery and obviously lacked the requisite dedication to my career (why would anyone want to go to business school?). However, I did return to work as planned, but now was armed with a fund of knowledge that neither he nor Dean Korn possessed. I had experienced a new world, one where profit, accountability, vibrancy, creativity, and merit counted. By comparison, academic surgery at Stanford, ruled by tradition and hierarchy, seemed dull, restrictive, and compromised.

Resuming my duties, I asked Dr. Hanbery to prepare the necessary papers and documentation required for promotion to full professor. Initially he demurred, telling me I had not published enough. I could not believe it. It turned out he was completely unaware of my laboratory's record of publication. Instead of drawing his attention to each and every paper I published (since he did not have the background in immunology to understand them), I had been content to update my vita on a regular basis, giving each revised copy to the departmental administrator, who dutifully filed it without comment. In contrast, I learned my male colleagues always prominently displayed a copy of each of their published papers on Hanbery's desk, where it could not escape his attention. Once he took a look at my vita Hanbery was convinced I deserved the promotion.

Gerry wrote a letter in support of the action, just as I had written a letter recommending his promotion two years before. Mine about Gerry was quite bland, ignoring any character issues, and had concentrated on his skills as a surgeon and teacher. One of the bizarre inconsistencies at academic medical centers is "confidential" information which rarely remains confidential, and the "honest" solicitation of opinion that is not expected to be entirely honest. Early in my career I wrote a letter supporting the promotion of an excellent anesthesiologist. It was extremely laudatory except for the statement "He is occasionally difficult to work with in the operating room." And he was! A flurry of letters and phone calls ensued asking what I had meant by the comment, would I rethink it, would I rewrite the letter please? I did.

I was the first woman to become a tenured full professor of neurosurgery in the United States. By this time Dr. Hanbery had developed into a strong advocate of mine, and took tremendous pride in my having "made it." Now instead of being teased, he received congratulations from his fellow program directors for having had the initiative to train and develop the career of one of the country's first female neurosurgeons. At the same time,

Gerry's attitude toward me, which had been fairly neutral since I joined the faculty, started to change in subtle ways.

Because of Dr. Hanbery's support, I had done my share of difficult cases and had developed a steady confidence in my surgical abilities. However, Gerry's behavior began subverting my position as "the surgeon." Sometime after my promotion I operated on a forty-five-year-old man at Stanford. Three weeks before, he had suffered a grand mal seizure for the first time ever. Epilepsy starting in this age group means a brain tumor until proven otherwise. The CT scan revealed an irregular white-rimmed doughnut, consistent in appearance with a highly malignant, rapidly growing cancer in the left anterior frontal lobe of his brain. Surgical resection would remove the vast majority of the lesion without undue risk of causing permanent paralysis of his right side or leaving him with disordered speech (the left side of the brain controls the right side of the body). Without surgery he would live a few months. With surgery, followed by radiation therapy to his brain, his range of life expectancy would be extended for nine to eighteen months. He had a daughter who was planning her wedding the following summer, and he was determined to walk her down the aisle.

An inexperienced but aggressive junior resident was working with me. He had scrubbed on only a few craniotomies in his nascent neurosurgical career and was thoroughly enjoying the chance to do a tumor case. For once, he was following my directions reasonably well, and I was not having to threaten him unduly. A piece of skull overlying the area of the tumor had been removed, and the dura (a thick, fibrous lining protecting the brain) had been incised and peeled back. I have a penchant for neatness during cranial surgery, and in spite of under-breath grumbles from the resident, he draped and clipped clean towels around the edges of the opening to the brain. The brain color was paler than the usual light salmon, and the normal wormlike gyral pattern was flattened; both observations indicated increased intracranial pressure. In the middle of the operative field the gyral pattern disappeared altogether, replaced by what looked like the top of a mushroom cloud from an atom bomb. The resident cauterized a small punctate area of brain surface in front of the abnormal area, and, following my verbal direction, was passing a hollow large-bore needle into the necrotic liquid center of the tumor. Suddenly, Gerry, laughing, noisily burst into the operating room and loudly asked me, "How's it going, honey?" All at once, I was no longer the neurosurgeon in charge. I had become one of his "honeys"—again. After looking at the tumor and telling the resident he was doing a good job, he left.

For a moment all work stopped and the only sounds in the room were from the respirator and the steady beep of the pulse monitor. "I don't know why he can't call me Fran," I finally said, breaking the silence. "I'm not his goddamned honey!" The circulating nurse, an older woman who had worked in the operating rooms from the time the hospital opened in 1959, and was of an age where she might have once changed Gerry's diapers, purred in a throaty voice, "That's O.K., he doesn't know my name either. If he didn't call me honey, I'd think he was sick." It took five minutes for me to reestablish a proper degree of control over the male resident—he had abruptly decided it was beneath him to work for a "honey." The remark also forced me to revisit the past, to return to my early days as a surgeon and ask myself, for what seemed like the millionth time, "Is a honey, especially *this* honey, good enough and talented enough to be doing this operation?" The patient not only escorted his daughter at her marriage but also lived to see his first grandchild.

I slowly began to understand that the combination of my academic title, a robust research program, and national recognition by fellow neurosurgeons (some of which was due to the fact that I was a woman) posed a considerable competitive threat to Gerry. He could not consider my training or functioning as a neurosurgeon to be of inferior quality to his. To do so would be self-criticism—we were both products of the same program, and he had taught me. Although he was two years ahead of me and had a full-time position at Stanford (I worked at the VA as well as at Stanford—an assignment with less prestige), Gerry chose gender as the means by which to establish his superior status. He defused my competitive threat by having our workplace acknowledge his male dominance, and more than ever before, "Fran" became "honey."

Yet at this point, I had never considered Gerry's behavior toward me as harassing. Harassment was something that happened to weak, vulnerable, younger women who did not have enough gumption to stand up for themselves. I was one tough hombre, too secure in my position and too mature to let myself be victimized. Gerry was simply part of that system that educated me, trained me, employed me, and toughened me, and nothing about that system was going to have a negative effect on *my* career. I had effectively insinuated myself into the cloistered world of academic neurosurgery and had proven I could make it. With Hanbery's presence, Gerry was like an annoying little gnat who could be brushed aside with the sweep of a hand. Despite the negative undercurrents from his running commentary I had earned the respect of our colleagues. All of us dismissed his off-the-cuff verbalizations as harmless.

Wrapped and totally immersed within the competitive cocoon of academic medicine, living every day at a great distance from the "real" world, I was all but oblivious to the fact that a woman's movement had started, and, selfishly, had no idea how other women in my own world were faring. I learned about that a couple of years later when what had been a low-key, almost hidden conflict exploded into open warfare.

3 When I joined the faculty in 1975, I knew Gerald Silverberg was the chair-elect for our department. He was Hanbery's personal choice, and over the years I never questioned that decision. Also, I had never thought much about what a switch from Jake to Gerry as chair would mean for the department and me. It is a human foible that, unrealistically, we assume our world will always be the same. Besides, I knew Gerry adored Dr. Hanbery and had watched him endeavor to become his clone. He adopted Hanbery's mannerisms, his pattern of speech, affected a pronounced limp similar to Hanbery's uneven gait, and even smoked a pipe for a few years. Blind loyalty had never allowed Hanbery to see or acknowledge any faults in his protégé, and he was steadfast in his support of him. Nevertheless, Gerry became increasingly restless about his own future around the time I was promoted to full professor.

By 1988 the department had added three neurosurgeons in junior faculty positions for a departmental total of six professionals. Two of the three additions had trained at Stanford, under the tutelage of Drs. Hanbery, Silverberg, and Conley. For years

Gerry had informed other neurosurgical program directors that he was personally responsible for the program's expansion and would be named chair at Stanford when Hanbery stepped down at age sixty-five. But Dr. Hanbery remained totally consumed by his brilliant practice, and had no interests apart from spending long hours at the hospital. He did not gracefully vacate the chair, as expected. Growing uneasy over Dr. Hanbery's continued presence and resiliency, fearful his own career as chair would be truncated, Gerry unleashed a vicious assault on Hanbery's character, deliberately reversing years of a very fast friendship and destroying a close mentor relationship.

All the details of what transpired remain sealed in documents from a closed court settlement. However, Hanbery's administrative assistant, Rose, was accused and eventually found guilty of misappropriating $285,000 of departmental funds. (The verdict was just: my name, for example, had been signed to restaurant receipts for meals I never ate, at times I could prove I had been in the operating room at the VA.) Gerry was the one who discovered the money was gone and notified the appropriate authorities. He had feuded bitterly with Rose for years (they were like two children vying for attention from their father) and took fiendish delight in exposing her thievery. But Dr. Hanbery, impeccably loyal, did not desert his longtime friend and helper, and supported her despite the cost to himself. After failing to separate Dr. Hanbery from Rose, Gerry also accused him of stealing money, and began building distance between himself and a potential scandal. He informed all who would listen (including patients waiting in examining rooms) that "the old fart" was failing as a surgeon and had, among other things, outlived his usefulness and robbed the department. At national meetings of neurosurgeons, I would be asked about what was happening at Stanford, and if it was really true that Gerry was going to be our next chair. Many wondered what had provoked the open conflict between Gerry and Jake. To those who would listen, Gerry boasted that under his stewardship the Stanford program would achieve the national academic prominence it richly deserved but had never attained because of its faulty leadership.

I was horrified by Gerry's persistent, invidious castigation of the chief. I realized Dr. Hanbery had his faults, but could not believe Gerry felt no loyalty whatever to the person who was most responsible for his academic position and success. More than once Dr. Hanbery wept bitterly in front of me, denying his personal involvement in the embezzlement, imploring me to tell him where he had gone wrong, and asking how his favorite "child" could turn on him so ferociously. Dr. Hanbery was totally bewildered and incredibly hurt. I felt I was being asked to play psychologist for one of the strongest people I had ever known—a person now reduced to a blathering, whimpering emptiness. Gerry was so sure he would be named the next chair, he, unbelievably, offered me the chance to join forces with him. He knew if both of us deserted him, Dr. Hanbery would be truly impotent. I was very angry and my answer to Gerry had been to "knock it off." I told him I found his actions truly appalling and completely unjustified, given all the unknowns in the money situation, as well as what he owed Dr. Hanbery for his years of support. Gerry later informed the confused residents and junior faculty, caught in the middle of this misery, that I was a total bitch. He also intimated orchestration on my part to thwart his deserved ascension to the departmental throne, and warned the others I was consumed by personal professional ambition.

One afternoon prior to starting my clinic, I was informed that two clerical staff members, Luann and Jolie, had just filed charges against Gerry alleging years of sexual harassment. I was very concerned about their welfare in the midst of the department turmoil, and asked them if they really understood the possible repercussions of their actions. They might have to answer embarrassing questions about their own pasts if anything were to come of their complaints, and they could expect significant retaliation from Gerry. The reality, at that point, was that Gerry would be, at the very least, the acting chair, and thus have control over their futures. Regardless of the outcome over the embezzlement charges, Dr. Hanbery would not maintain his leadership position, because of his lack of oversight over departmental finances. The two women remained resolute, and vehemently denied that Dr. Hanbery had, in any way, suggested or encouraged their grievances. Jolie and Luann would stay, they told me, until and if Dr. Hanbery left. Their accusations were based on hard facts, and they wanted Gerry's behavior toward them, and others, to change.

I was amazed, and, at the same time, frightened for them. For years I had watched Gerry revel in his reputation as a consummate womanizer, acting out even in front of patients who not only heard his remarks but also witnessed his blatantly seductive manner with numerous secretaries in the clinic area as well as with nurses on the floor. But no matter how inappropriate his behavior was, no one ever before had considered Gerry to be guilty of actually harassing anyone—he was a bit outlandish, more than a little childish, but he was part of the culture and most labeled him a case of arrested maturity who was often quite funny. Following my colleagues' advice, I had never confronted him and that was my recommendation to Luann and Jolie after my brief conversation with them.

Gerry's pressure tactics worked. Dr. Hanbery resigned the chairmanship amid many questions about his own personal integrity. He was eventually exonerated of any wrong, and received a letter of apology from the university for the accusations originating with Gerry. Although he was named to the emeritus professoriate, Dr. Hanbery shunned the university and established a small private consultative practice, absenting himself from all contact with the medical school. As everyone expected, a few weeks after Dr. Hanbery's resignation, in mid-1989, Dean Korn named Dr. Gerald Silverberg acting chair of the Department of Neurosurgery.

At about the same time, after a hiatus of twelve years, I was again elected chair of the Medical Faculty Senate, and thus was once again a member of the dean's Executive Committee. Gerry too joined this powerful group when he became acting chair. Except for the recent commotion in my department, I was quite happy with my day-to-day life and interacted easily with professional colleagues and patients.

But what I had not previously realized was the degree to which Dr. Hanbery had been responsible for creating an environment in which I, as a woman, could flourish. He had three daughters, and in some ways I became his fourth, and ultimately he wanted me to succeed. His presence made it possible for me to ignore my colleagues, including Gerry, and pay no attention to whatever little sexist power games were being played.

When Dr. Hanbery had been around, Gerry and I treated each other with restraint. We were not the best of friends. I found his arrogance, his boasting and overt sexism intolerable and his subtle, but increasing objections to my presence were known to many. But we were both adults and professionals and made the necessary effort to coexist with an outward appearance of relative harmony—so much so that one of our colleagues asked Gerry and me to operate together to remove a ruptured disk from his back.

But when Gerry was appointed acting chair, the sunshine left my world. Like a feudal baron, he triumphantly established his castle in Dr. Hanbery's large, recently vacated office. His first move was to send the office couch to the dry cleaners. Gerry was certain that shortly he would be named permanent chair and began using the absolute power that the academic world confers on its executive appointees. Prior to Dr. Hanbery's departure, he had mercilessly been picking on one of our new assistant professors, a man hired by Dr. Hanbery, and someone Gerry did not like. In a terribly misguided attempt to be funny, Gerry, with mock humor and horror, repeatedly and relentlessly called him a "murderer" when he had a less than ideal surgical result with a patient. With his appointment Gerry's criticism became louder, more frequent, and had greater authority, so that residents, when possible, avoided working with the young neurosurgeon, and the nursing and clerical staffs genuinely believed he was dangerous. He was not—he did some cases at the VA and had very acceptable and occasionally spectacular surgical results. Gerry rapidly destroyed the remainder of his career at Stanford, and within a few months of Gerry's being named acting chair, he left for another academic position.

Gerry now also controlled my work environment and he wasted no time distancing me from others in the department. For years the VA and Stanford had shared grand rounds and conferences, and the resident assigned to the VA moved freely between the two institutions. By fiat all combined rounds moved to Mecca (Stanford), and Gerry separated the VA from Stanford as if all our patients carried the plague and the resident and I who worked there were likewise infected. The other faculty member assigned to the VA began, with Gerry's encouragement, spending more of his time at Stanford. The bewildered resident stationed at the VA was stranded when his stream of information about events at Stanford was truncated. Initially, I thought Gerry was merely testing his recently acquired authority, and was not too surprised since I had been so openly critical of his treatment of Dr. Hanbery. With time, I expected, my life would return to normal. But as the VA program became increasingly isolated from Stanford, my suspicions and unhappiness escalated, and I began to think I too might be more welcome and content at another institution.

In the wake of disruption and ugliness surrounding Dr. Hanbery's departure, a number of office and clinic personnel, including Luann and Jolie, quit rather than work for Gerry, so my relations with the Stanford staff changed. Overnight, the climate for me turned icy. New people had been hired by Gerry and, as their boss, he came first. It's not that they were deliberately negative. They were just detached from me, realizing I had no say in their job description, promotions, or pay.

A number of incidents confirmed my sense that I was considered a lesser being. In midafternoon one day I finished seeing a patient, and walked down the clinic hallway to the open waiting/

reception area. Three of my patients were sitting amid the plastic potted palms and ficus trees. I picked up a chart and called the first patient. Then I felt a restraining hand on my arm.

"There aren't any rooms free right now, Doctor," the clinic nurse said to me.

"Why not?"

"Even though it's not his clinic day, Dr. Silverberg scheduled two patients for this afternoon and told me to put them in rooms as soon as they got here. They both arrived at once, so they're in your rooms. Sorry." In Dr. Hanbery's time, the nurse would have asked my permission before unilaterally filling the examination rooms with Gerry's patients and making mine wait.

On another day I was in an examining room with a patient and we both heard a knock on the door. Before I could get to the door, it opened, and Gerry poked his head in and said to me, "Hon, can you come into my office for a minute?" My immediate reaction was, what's this poor patient going to think? Are we having an affair? How can a patient take me seriously as a neurosurgeon if he or she thinks I am one of Gerry's honeys and am willing to play with him during office hours?

Gerry was aware we had differences we should try to resolve. Many times I sat in his office at his invitation—hardly a neutral location, but appropriate and not particularly uncomfortable for me given that he was the acting chair. But time and again we would barely have begun a dialogue to address the pressing problem of the moment when he would abruptly declare that he was unable to continue the conversation. Then he would ask me to join him for dinner, or a drink, or lunch to finish our discussion. The next day his secretary would phone my office at the VA, often multiple times, to find a mutually agreeable date and time and place.

It was hard to believe we could not just talk like two normal human beings. But I was frankly uncomfortable with the thought of going elsewhere and managed to avoid all of his invitations using a succession of contrived, but creative excuses. In retrospect

I should have told him up front I would not go out with him in public, and why. I realize now had I been a good team player, I would have made an effort to meet Gerry outside of our workplace, if only to provide an environment that was more comfortable and communicative for *him*. But when the agenda itself concerns power, there is no such thing as a free lunch, and my psyche had only so much resiliency.

Of course I accept invitations from male colleagues—when I feel good about *me* when I am with *them*. Over the years some of the younger "old guard" of neurosurgeons mellowed and realized that at least a few women were there to stay. Many have become good friends of mine, and most have been extremely helpful in guiding and building my career on a national level. At professional meetings we go out, ever mindful that malicious gossip from our colleagues may ensue—something we brush off. I am respected by these men, and regardless of any power differential between us, they have no need to establish dominance. I trust my instincts enough to know that if I am uneasy in a social setting with male professionals, there is something wrong with the relationship, and the wrong usually is that man's attempt or need to diminish me in some way.

Evening rounds became Gerry's show time for the residents, interns, and students. He was determined to establish his dominance over all, and be viewed as the absolute kingpin of neurosurgeons. Gerry never seemed to realize that as he ascended the academic ladder to become a full professor and acting chair, his comments were taken more seriously than they had been when he was an intern. The academic environment, and probably especially in surgery, where good and bad can be measured by patient outcome, is one that breeds a game of destructive criticism. The game is played by most of its inhabitants, including yours truly. But it is criticism which is usually contained and heard by only a few well-chosen ears. Gerry played this game very differently from most of us, willingly embellishing the entire hospital with his critical voice, without thought or concern as to how far his message reached or who received it.

Gerry openly criticized not only his own faculty but also physicians outside our department. Our group would periodically visit tiny babies with brain hemorrhages in the neonatal intensive care unit. In a voice heard by everyone, including nurses and anxious parents hovering over their tiny baby's incubator, Gerry would inform his attentive entourage that pediatricians were not really very bright (that's why they went into pediatrics). Especially dull were those pediatricians electing to work with premature infants—so-called doctors who knew nothing more than how to shove a breathing tube down tiny windpipes. He trivialized concerns nurses had about their patients, telling them, poor dears, they had no ability to figure out what was really important. His insensitivity even extended to the patient. One day, at the bedside of an immobile, dying patient, a young girl with an inoperable brain-stem tumor, Gerry said with a silly laugh that there was nothing to do because she was going to die. Outside the patient's room, the nurse assigned to the case reminded Gerry that the patient could hear and understand everything. He told the nurse he didn't care.

In late fall 1989, my problems with Gerry took an ominous turn. It became obvious that having tenure would not guarantee a productive work environment or one where I would be happy. I started making inquiries about academic positions elsewhere. What happened during our department's annual search for a new resident further confirmed my inclination to leave.

Our residency program takes one new resident each year, and until the early 1980s that choice had been made unilaterally by Dr. Hanbery. Now all of the faculty participate in the selection process. Residency positions in neurosurgery are extremely competitive, as there are only a limited number of training programs in the United States. The discipline attracts the most intelligent graduating medical students. Because of Stanford's overall reputation our neurosurgery program receives applications from the most talented of an already elite group. Every fall we review over a hundred applications for our one open position. The idea is to identify and attract the one best-qualified resident who will benefit the most from the strengths of our particular program. At Stanford, our program has a reputation for its superb clinical training—almost all of our graduates (except those who have remained at Stanford) have gone into private practice, rather than stay in academics. Ours is not known as a program with a strong research focus where a resident gets extensive research experience along with training in neurosurgery. Thus, an applicant wholly committed to an academic career, where building a future research program is expected, gains more legitimacy for such a career if he or she were to graduate from a program designed to train academicians, rather than pure clinicians.

In the early weeks of the resident selection process for 1989, the faculty reviewed folders and winnowed the number of possible candidates. I was reminded that nothing much had changed in gender relations in my profession by a letter of recommendation for a female applicant written by a well-known program director. He wrote, "This young lady spent a month on the neurosurgery service based at the VA hospital. She is an above-average individual who is pleasant, courteous, honest, and shows no psychotic behavior. She is clearly pleasantly aggressive and was always available to help out in both the OR and on the floor." Pleasant, courteous, fortunately not psychotic. But what can she do? How did she perform? In past years I had ignored the lukewarm nature of letters written about female resident candidates, but against a backdrop of my own escalating career problems with Gerry, this letter signaled to me that sexism in medical schools was very much alive—and potentially harmful.

Fourth-year medical student Anton Stevens arrived from Harvard in our first interview group in 1989. An exceptionally well-qualified candidate, he could hardly contain his infectious enthusiasm for the Stanford program. For the past two years of medical school he had been working with Dr. Lily Louis, a basic science researcher whose work explored, on a molecular level, how white blood cells migrated from the circulation into the brain. The pathology of a number of neurologic diseases, for example, multiple sclerosis and viral encephalitis, is defined by the presence of these immunologically active white blood cells in brain tissue—in the normal brain, they are absent. The antitumor effect developed in my laboratory also depended on white blood cells migrating to the brain in response to an injected stimulus. Thus, the work from our two laboratories was quite interrelated and Lily and I had met at scientific conferences in the past on a few occasions.

Anton Stevens had already decided Stanford would be his first choice of neurosurgery programs because he could continue his Harvard work in my laboratory. While he was very interested in developing good surgical skills, he envisioned his future in an academic setting. It was fun to talk with someone who spoke my research language, but I cautioned Anton that my laboratory should not be the primary factor in his decision about which training program would be best for him. "It's possible," I warned, "this laboratory and I won't be here when you're ready for your year in the lab. Look carefully at all the other elements of our program. We all take great pride in training very good operating neurosurgeons, but if you really want an academic career, that may not be enough."

In addition, Anton and I talked about hazards for residents joining programs without a permanent chair. He asked for my prediction of Stanford's future. "If I had to guess, I believe Dr. Silverberg will be appointed chair—unfortunately. I say that because I don't think he's the best person to head this program, and I'm not sure he'll support my continuing research effort. If he becomes permanent chair, I'll most likely leave and my laboratory will cease to exist. I'm really hoping someone from the outside gets the job and establishes Stanford as an academic training center, but we sure aren't there now. Our two new assistant professors are just beginning to get their acts together and mine's the only lab really going—in fact, one of them's actually working in my lab with me now. Unfortunately, the dean hasn't started any search, and I'm not sure if or when he intends to do so."

That evening, I stopped at Stanford Hospital to see two patients, then went to the department office to pick up mail. Gerry had just locked his office to go home for the night, and was fifty feet down the hall from me on his way to the parking lot. He heard me unlock the main office door, turned around, then yelled at me that he did not want me to see any more resident candidates—that I was hindering his ability to sell the program. (For prestige value and to build his own ego, he was marketing our program as one that produced academic neurosurgeons.)

I knew exactly what had happened. During his interview with Gerry, Anton Stevens had expressed disappointment over the possibility there might be no research position with me in the future, and had asked some penetrating questions about leadership. Gerry made no effort to lessen the physical distance between us by walking back toward me. "You mean you want me to lie?" I shouted back.

Having no trouble being heard, Gerry responded that I was much too negative and my negative views were preventing him from getting the best man (sic) for the program. Talking over the fifty feet that still separated us, I told him he was not being fair, that I was entitled to my opinion, and the kids deserved an honest appraisal, especially if he was giving them an overly optimistic, and essentially inaccurate, picture. He retorted I had damned our program with faint praise, and from now on was off the interview schedule.

I could not believe what I was hearing. Possibly I had been more critical than necessary about our program, but I wanted to be candid and open with the students about the environment they would be coming into. I frankly could not visualize any dazzling future for Stanford as an academic center if Gerry was named its permanent chair. He may have been deeply offended by hearing this. In my defense, it was not fair for a student to assume he or she could work with me if I was about to leave. Perhaps I should have been more moderate in my presentation, but I, too, can be a difficult person—opinionated, outspoken, self-confident, and painfully blunt.

Yet despite my shortcomings, Gerry had no right to dictate what I could or could not say during an interview. Further, he had no right to limit my functioning as a faculty member, especially since I was a tenured full professor. I immediately tried to resolve the impasse. "Why don't you schedule things so you always have the exit interview? You're the acting chair here, they're going to believe you, not me. If you're the last one they see, you can easily undo any damage you think I've done. You'll have the final word and impression. Tell them I'm negative, bitchy, miserable, hard to work with, not a team player, whatever—but I'm not going to change what I'm saying—I'm telling the truth about this program."

Without any hesitation Gerry again told me I was out. Seething, he turned abruptly and, limping, rapidly walked away. And out I was. At the time I was the only one who dared to be openly critical of Gerry—none of the others had tenure.

At a national meeting of neurosurgeons in 1990, a program director asked me why I had not interviewed two very good students from his medical school who were looking at our program. I told him about the prohibition and asked for his thoughts. He answered, "Part of Gerry's agenda is to keep you hidden so he can shine. You're far more visible than he is—you've done more—and his goddamn ego just can't put up with that. It's really very simple." Tenure provided no protection from this type of hierarchical abuse—not in a medical school where executive leadership positions are conferred for an academic lifetime. An ancient but flawed system protected Gerry, and he had lots of company in other divisional and departmental chairs at Stanford. A chair, or acting chair, has enough power to limit, even destroy, any member of his department. The department or division leader controls such resources as research space, operating time, secre-

tarial support, and financial remuneration. Unless there is organized, total revolt by a division or department, a chair's behavior
is not usually open to overt, well-founded criticism or questioning
by individual faculty. Gripes are voiced clandestinely and injustices suffered silently. Otherwise, a career is ruined. The only
thing Gerry could not do was to terminate my employment. So
my only hope for survival at Stanford was that the dean not give
power to him on a permanent basis.

By now I was convinced that he was not suitable for an extended period of executive leadership in which people would be
treated fairly. I was also aware I was the only faculty member
who was in a position to question behavior that I saw as increasingly inappropriate and embarrassing to the department. Proac-
tively I initiated a mini crusade, without real structure or specific
focus, except to question his leadership potential, something I felt
I had every right to do.

Six months after Gerry became acting chair, I shared my anx-
ieties in two separate, miserably uncomfortable half-hour sessions, first with the university president and then the dean of the
medical school. I talked to each in general terms and labeled none
of the outstanding issues "sexist," although I did tell them in
general terms I thought Gerry's actions around women were not
always proper. I doubt either administrator would have understood a charge of sexism or sexual harassment. Neither could
have known that Luann and Jolie had already filed sexual harassment charges against Gerry: grievances brought by members
of the staff are handled by the hospital, not the medical school
or university.

Instead, what the president and dean heard were my thoughts
about Gerry's inadequate leadership skills and behavioral deviancy: what happens when power is defined one dimensionally as
power over others, that he destroyed people rather than built
them. Each man listened politely, but from a distance, and at the
end of his session the president passed the baton to the dean.
Although I do not remember his exact words, the dean essentially

told me not to worry my pretty little head. He also promptly informed Gerry that I had paid him a visit.

Going to work each day became an unenjoyable chore, especially days when I had to work at Stanford when my stomach pH would turn very acidic. Although they remained friendly with me, the three junior faculty declared allegiance to Gerry. It was required for their academic survival. I found departmental faculty meetings very difficult, but I had to attend, as they were my only source of information. Everyone was aware there was significant antagonism between Gerry and me. Any suggestion I made was immediately negated by Gerry, even if supported by the others. I began using Dr. Joe Andrus, who spent part time at the VA with me, as my emissary. My ideas would be funneled through his voice, and that way they would, at least, be considered and discussed. After one particularly nasty, contentious meeting, Joe told me how Gerry, after I left, began ranting in a loud voice, heard by the entire office and clinic staff, that PMS had to be the primary reason for my being such a difficult person.

I knew Gerry wanted me gone from Stanford—I had not kissed his ring in loyal allegiance, I held him responsible for destroying the end of Dr. Hanbery's illustrious career, and I am sure the dean had shared with him my reservations about his leadership qualities. Instead of using the authority of his position to help build and strengthen the neurosurgery program at the VA, because it was my program and my research laboratories he worked through fear and intimidation to destroy them—and, with them, me. Phil and I both felt I was dying a slow death, one that was inevitable and one we had no control over. I was so unhappy that I began to look seriously at a few jobs, upon invitation, at other academic institutions. I declined one offer extended by a good friend and neurosurgical program director in the East, because there was no developed laboratory space and I would have to reestablish my complicated research enterprise from the very beginning.

I was also invited to explore two positions as chair of a neurosurgical program, and would have accepted one had it been offered. In my travels, I found the academic world not quite ready for its first-ever female chair of a department or division of neurosurgery. In academic medicine, I learned, tokenism has become prevalent in job searches. A friend who runs her own executive search firm told me instructions from academic institutions often indirectly suggest she supply a list of candidates and include one person of color and one woman, making certain they cannot qualify for the job. Most universities now mandate an affirmative action component to any search. So long as a woman (white) and a person of color (either gender) has been *identified* for the particular position, affirmative action guidelines are satisfied. More points are scored, however, if the candidate actually visits and, after interviews and a seminar presentation, is found to be "not exactly what we're looking for." When one is the token, tokenism is easy to recognize. A faculty member from the institution with the chair position I would have accepted told me some months later that had I been male, the job would have been offered to me, as I was the most qualified candidate they had interviewed.

After unrewarding attempts, spanning many months, to find a suitable position away from Stanford at a location that was acceptable to Phil, I started asking myself, why should I be forced to relinquish all I had accomplished? Why should I leave my friends, my contacts, my laboratory, my patients? Phil really did not want to move, and neither of us could envision a commuter marriage. He was angry I was being drummed out of the corps without cause, by the actions of a single individual. The rest of the university apparently embraced me. I was elected to the University Advisory Board, the highest-ranking faculty committee for the entire university. It was a distinct honor. In 1990 I was re-elected chair of the Medical Faculty Senate. These positions gave me monthly contact with the president and provost of the university, involvement at the highest level of decision making, and access to very important information. With such widespread recognition within Stanford, why should I leave?

Academic life at Stanford changed quite abruptly in 1990. Research money from governmental sources rapidly slowed to a barely perceptible trickle. Stanford had been accused of using grant money to pay for yachts, silk sheets, and its president's wedding reception. An arcane pooled accounting system had led to slack, almost lackadaisical oversight over money, and no one knew which funds were paying for what, when, or how much. When the university indignantly declared its innocence, the government responded by withdrawing financial support, requesting repayment, and raising the possibility of punitive sanctions which, if levied, could cost the university in excess of $200 million. The government also drastically cut the reimbursement rate for indirect costs associated with research (costs of water, electricity, gas, depreciation), presenting the university and its medical school with an unexpected $40 million deficit for 1991. Although the entire university, of necessity, began cutting costs wherever possible, the medical school was the most affected unit.

Financial experts quickly turned to clinical doctors, those who care for patients as their primary endeavor within the medical school. These physicians also make money, and if given resources to increase the number of patients seen, could make more. Unlike research dollars coming from grants, clinical income is derived from examining patients, doing operations, taking X-rays, performing diagnostic tests, and generating and sending bills for services rendered—just like doing business in the real world. The urgent message from health care economists was that a rapid switch in source of income was essential for the survival of the Stanford Medical School.

Our clinical faculty is quite specialized, taking great pride in being able to do radical, complex procedures and treat the most refractory diseases with newly discovered treatment protocols. But the viability of highly trained tertiary care physicians (those doing, for example, heart transplants and joint replacements, or treating complex cases of leukemia) depends on a constant stream of patient referrals from primary care doctors. And there was only a rudimentary primary care base among those on the clinical faculty. Such mundane medicine had always been beneath the dignity of the institution. Patients sought Stanford; it had never been the other way around.

Dean David Korn failed to heed warnings about the economic clout of health maintenance organizations and their increasing ability to control access to patients. In order to retain control of the medical school and protect erosion of his research power base, he rejected alliances with the Palo Alto and Menlo Medical Clinics, both well-regarded community health care providers. Such partnerships, it turned out, would have been advantageous to all and given Stanford the well-established primary care units it needed. As it was, faculty hours of work per week increased, collections for provided services decreased, cost-of-living allowances died, and the medical school became a fiscal burden to the university. Like a rapidly moving weather front, changes in the health care system engulfed the medical center and brought wind and rain before a shielding umbrella could be opened. Many held the dean responsible for the lack of shelter. Additionally, one of the most profitable units, the Department of Neurosurgery, still had no permanent chair, and no search had been started. David Korn could have recruited a visible, high-powered academic clinician for the post, telegraphing to the rest of the medical school that he recognized the need for building first-class clinical, rather than basic, research programs. To do so, however, would have been a true departure from the way he had operated in the past.

David Korn is a fascinating combination of intellectual brilliance, political savvy, and narrowness of scope. He is a pathologist. Thus his practice of medicine never included interaction with live patients. As chair of his department and later as dean, his mandate was to build a research and clinical laboratory powerhouse. It was his job to find research money. As he saw his deanship tarnished by momentous financial crisis, the government funding scandal, and a health care revolution in which patients became top priority, he became increasingly insular, defining his world by the four walls of his office. His insularity is best symbolized by a wall. Until his tenure, students could enter the dean's office by any of three doors, one of which connected the Office of Student Affairs with the dean's executive suite. After David became dean, a permanent wall was installed between the offices. Students now used the other entrances only in response to a formal summons. At graduation, in a moment of idle curiosity, I asked a medical student what he thought of his dean. He replied, "The dean? What dean? Only time I ever saw him was when he talked to us on orientation day four years ago."

David was simply not attuned to the human dimension of medicine. There were many other physicians at Stanford who were equally ill equipped, and harboring populations of such doctors may be a problem encountered by academic medical centers in general. For academicians, humanity takes time, rarely leads to personal glory, and does not pay the bills. I believe the dean considered it someone else's job to teach humanity to the medical community. His department chairs did not have that responsibility either, and his choice of chairs, as well as his method for choosing them, reflected that bias. All executive positions had to be ratified by the Executive Committee, but the action was always pro forma. David chose his chairs on the basis of how beholden they would be to him. Powerful, charismatic individuals, more often than not, were eliminated from consideration. Clinical chairs were left vacant for years. The dean seemed content to watch the leaderless units falter and become moribund so that he, as a knight in shining armor, could rescue them.

There are some prominent examples of this phenomenon. In early 1988, after a loud verbal altercation which was the culmination of four years of differing opinions, Dean Korn abruptly fired his chair of the Department of Surgery. It was not until late 1990, two search committees and many talented candidates later, that a successor was chosen from the rubble. By this time the

Department of Surgery had lost every vestige of power and respect it once held in the medical school and among departments
of surgery nationally.

Also in 1988, a faculty search committee worked diligently for
many months to find a new chair for the Radiology Department,
and had identified the top leaders in the field who might accept
the position at Stanford. Dean Korn requested a slate of candidates. However, his favored son was not on the final list. So the
dean thanked the search committee for their efforts and informed
them, by letter, that he was appointing his desired candidate,
whom the committee had considered and rejected. The committee
was outraged. They had wasted many hours of valuable time on
a process they had never controlled. A year later, after a disagree-
ment with the chair of the Ophthalmology Department, Dean
Korn unilaterally dismissed him and replaced him on a permanent
basis with another faculty member without conducting any search
whatever.

Then in March 1991, almost two years after Gerry's interim
appointment, with the medical school in unstable fiscal circumstances, Dean Korn announced to the faculty he had established
a search committee for our department chair. In his charge to the
committee the dean asked for a slate of names, as opposed to one
finalist, and suggested they consider, as appropriate, qualified inside candidates.

I was ecstatic. Gerry was visibly shaken by the news. He had
been waiting two years to move from acting to permanent chair,
and fully expected to be appointed in the absence of a search and
any review of his qualifications.

On a rainy day in late March, I met briefly with the search
committee at one of their first organizational gatherings. It was
held in the dean's conference room, a poorly lighted place ru-
mored by some to be wired for surveillance purposes. Wind had
blown rain toward the windows, filling the tiny steel squares of
exterior screening with water, converting the screens into visual
shields that hid the outside world and made the dark room even

darker. The discussion was candid. Because of the university's budget problems, two outside consultants, both neurosurgery program directors at other medical schools, had visited Stanford a few months earlier to advise the dean about the search. Recognizing we needed a national presence, both had strongly recommended going outside for a leader. They were certain the Stanford name would draw an excellent collection of candidates, despite obvious institutional financial constraints.

Committee members and I discussed the composition, focus, and academic mission of the department. I told them we needed an infusion of new blood because four of the five of us had graduated from our own program. I believe our residents are hurt by not having wider exposure to different ways of taking care of neurosurgical problems, and should learn that the Stanford way is not the only way. I knew a number of talented neurosurgeons who not only were interested in the position but also would bring immediate luster to our program. The committee chair, Dr. Lance Dickenson, asked me for names. I gave him four without hesitation, and promised more after doing some thinking.

"Do you want the job?" I was asked. My response was careful. "I believe I'm qualified for the job and have the right balance of clinical work vs. research, but it wouldn't work, not with what's happened in the department since the Hanbery mess. So, no. I'm not a candidate and don't want to be considered. Find us someone good, someone who can put us on the map. All the elements of an outstanding program are here; we just need someone to pull it together for us."

Then they asked the really tough question. How would the department do with Gerry as chair?

I dared not say what I really thought. I had no idea whether any in this group were beholden to Gerry or had already promised him their support. My life was difficult enough, and if an outside person was chosen, Gerry and I would continue to be faculty members in the same small department, with a need to be civil to one another. There was no good reason to escalate the animosity by raising the specter of his embarrassing and sexist behavior. My future was critically dependent on their finding a neurosurgeon from another institution, someone with good leadership skills, someone willing to accept me as a member of the faculty based on my credentials, irrespective of my gender. So I spoke cautiously. "While he's an excellent teacher and a very good surgeon, I don't believe he knows how to make people—if you will—'all they can be.' And I don't think he has a clue about what a research program really entails—he's just never played the game." Our conversation moved to other topics—strengths and weaknesses of the other faculty, clinical programs of the future, additions to the departmental research base. My meeting with them lasted approximately twenty minutes.

As I opened the far door to leave, I turned back to the group, and in parting told them, "I think you would hear the same from Gerry about me, but if he's the best you can do, I'll resign and leave Stanford."

Over the next two months the search committee received more than thirty résumés from neurosurgeons across the United States who were interested in the Stanford program. Many were distinguished, active physicians who could bring national prominence, as well as established sources of both clinical and research revenue to the department, the school, and the dean's office.

On Wednesday, May 22, 1991, without prior notification to his search committee and without their approval, Dean Korn abruptly halted the search.

4 I remember the early evening of May 22, 1991, as if it were yesterday. Before heading home at the end of a long day, I had traveled from the VA to Stanford to see a patient in the intensive care unit. Mrs. Rawls had suffered an extensive brain hemorrhage two days before. Because the bleed inside her head had been so large and so destructive, a decision had been made by her family and me to do nothing surgically. No one expected her to survive. But she had been placed on life support because a son and a daughter were en route to say a formal goodbye, and the family had asked me to try to keep her alive until they arrived. The junior neurosurgical resident had drilled a small hole in her skull and directed a catheter into her right lateral ventricle to drain spinal fluid, relieving the malignant pressure that would have quickly ended her life. So fifty-six hours later, Mrs. Rawls, essentially "brain dead," technically was still alive.

When I walked into the intensive care unit (ICU) she was propped up in bed at a twenty-degree angle. Her upper body was uncovered, breasts exposed and pasted with EKG pads. Traces of talcum powder, recently applied, dusted both armpits and the skin underneath her breasts. Her eyes were taped shut, and were the only part of her face left undisturbed. Tubes seemed to come out of, or were attached, everywhere else—from nose, mouth, ears, and even her head. Part of her scalp had been shaved and a tube exiting through a gauze dressing was filled with pink fluid, a combination of blood and spinal fluid. A respirator breathed for her and was but one of many machines maintaining and monitoring her vital functions.

I had not known Mrs. Rawls when she had been truly alive. I knew she had a brain problem my skill as a surgeon could not correct, and thus kept an emotional distance from her—something every doctor learns to do, especially when a patient's life is beyond hope. The tube draining fluid from her brain had plugged up, and I should have just left it that way and not prolonged the inevitable. But by a reflex reaction belonging to every neurosurgeon, I asked for a syringe of saline so I could clear it. As I was unplugging the line, my beeper went off. I removed my gloves, pushed the recall button, and saw a telephone extension number I did not recognize. Suddenly I became quite apprehensive. I penned my required daily "No Code" order on the order sheet—when and if Mrs. Rawls's heart stopped, there was to be no effort made to restart it—and left the room, closing the sliding glass door behind me.

There were numerous phones on the triangular desk work area of the ICU. Wanting privacy, I picked up the receiver of one at a distance from the unit clerk and two nurses who were working on charts. I punched in the number and was startled to hear "Good afternoon, this is the dean's office."

"I hope his secretary's getting paid overtime" nonsensically flashed through my mind. "This is Dr. Conley, I'm answer . . ."

The secretary interrupted. "Oh yes, thank you for calling. Dean Korn was most anxious to reach you this evening." I could feel my heart rate accelerating. Somehow I knew what was coming.

The dean's voice is very familiar to me, as I have known him for as long as I have been on the faculty. But the man on the phone did not sound like him. His words were strangled, as if each were escaping the confines of a voice box stuffed with cotton and shoved into being by willpower alone. He told me that because of the school's money situation, he had just called off the national search and would appoint Professor Silverberg to be chair of the department. He added he hoped to announce his decision sometime in the coming week. The message confirmed vague rumors that had been circulating for the past few days.

I struggled to answer him and heard my voice as if it came from a great, echoing distance and from someone other than me. He had the right to know I had heard his message, along with all of its implications. "Well, I'm very disappointed, as you have to know, but I do appreciate your taking the time and trouble to tell me before you make the official announcement. You'll have my resignation notice on your desk in the morning."

The dean had now recovered most of his normal voice. The difficult part of this conversation was over for him. "I hope you'll reconsider and think carefully . . ."

"All the necessary thinking has been done over these past two years, David. I've already written my resignation. I just need to retrieve it from the computer. You'll have it in the morning." The words connected fluently, the result of multiple past silent rehearsals. Suddenly I felt so angry, so defeated, and so crushed, tears filled my eyes. I hoped no one was watching.

"I'm sorry . . ."

"So am I." We both hung up, and I walked out of the ICU staring at the ground so the tears would fall there instead of running down my face.

As I walked to the parking lot, I was overwhelmed by a profound sense of betrayal. I sat in my car and let the tears flow freely. My decision to resign was not based on academic politics or on basic personality differences although I am sure the dean viewed it that way. I, who thought I could not be touched by political infighting, who was secure in my own world, even arrogant, had just become a symbol defining the state of our academic medical system, certainly at Stanford, and most probably at other medical schools as well. The fact that Dean David Korn *would* appoint as chair of my department someone who expressed an overt contempt for women, and lacked the basic fundamentals of humanity, was a direct, hard slap to my face, and confirmed, in a manner vivid enough for all to see, my second-class citizenship within our work environment.

The next day, Thursday, was the only day of the workweek I had no assigned patient care activities after routine morning hospital rounds. Thursdays were my "lab" days. They began in the early daylight with the same five a.m. alarm as on any other weekday, but instead of the nonstop hurry of other mornings, they proceeded in slow motion. My daily run on dirt trails in the adjacent park was always a little longer, a little less compulsive—a more joyous experience. Most mornings, drinking a mug of coffee and fixing my hair were simultaneous activities; Thursdays, I could do them one at a time. On that particular Thursday in late May my early run was considerably more contemplative than usual, and before leaving for work, I actually sat at the dining-room table and, bathed by a sharp-edged, oblique ray of morning sunshine coming through the glass door, combined coffee with a luxurious, thorough reading of the entire morning paper. A future life without the hassle of getting ready for work every day seemed very enticing.

When I reached my office at the VA, I turned on my computer and scrolled the contents of documents to "resign note." A year or so before, I had written a resignation notice in a moment of pique, after a particularly contentious faculty meeting. I was testing the experience, somehow knowing the note would be needed in the future. After changing and updating it, I printed it on a piece of departmental stationery and drove the few miles to the medical center to deliver it personally to Dean Korn, who was occupied behind the heavy door of his office. I left the notice with his secretary.

It was dated May 23 and read:

Dear David:

Per our phone conversation last evening this letter will serve as official notification of resignation of my position at Stanford University School of Medicine as a Professor of Neurosurgery, effective 1 September 1991. For the past two years my working environment at the School of Medicine has been less than ideal and your appointment of Gerald Silverberg to the position of chairman of the department and cessation of a national search for the position indicate that change to a less hostile environment for me will not be forthcoming as I had hoped. I am sure you will agree that life is too short to live it in misery!

Stanford has always been an institution that has striven for excellence—your decision demonstrates your willingness to accept less than that. I do appreciate your notifying me about your decision prior to its general dissemination.

Sincerely,
Frances K. Conley, M.D.

I had signed the letter simply "Fran" and sent a copy to the university president, Donald Kennedy.

I knew others in our medical community had objections to the appointment of Gerry as chair of the Department of Neurosurgery, but doubted any would dare challenge the dean over his choice. Once I departed, the dean's appointment would be accomplished smoothly and without rancor, and the Neurosurgery Department would stabilize, erasing two years of chronic irritation for him.

I drove back to the VA to meet with my laboratory group. I

remember the day as full of bright sunshine with little fluffy white clouds casting dark moving smudges on the blond foothills behind the campus. Instead of despondency over the end of a high-profile career, I was feeling exhilarated at the thought of freedom from its daily burdens. Suddenly I acquired an uncanny, enhanced ability to appreciate the physical beauty of California in late spring. It was as if a dark gray cloak, worn every day of my professional life for the past two years, suddenly blazed in Technicolor, and, as it was whirled off, I was tossed spinning into the "real" world, where I was welcomed, for the first time ever, as an active participant. My past status as physician spectator was forgiven and forgotten. I could not wait to get out from under, to really live, to do something different, although I did not know what. The only career I had ever known was "academic neuro-surgeon"—would that I had the voice to sing opera, the artistic talent to make movies, the perseverance to pursue a Ph.D. in philosophy. I looked up at the sky and laughed with the sun.

Unfortunately, my brief bout of expansive euphoria soon passed and Thursday then continued as usual. At 10 a.m. in my large downstairs laboratory, my group of students and postdocs had gathered in a rough circle of haphazard chairs and stools. Surrounding them on laboratory counters and tables were microscopes, glass staining dishes, cryostats, a tissue processor, and stacked cardboard trays of tissue sample vials, each with visible remnants of a rodent brain resting in formalin. In one corner were neat stacks of white paraffin tissue blocks waiting to be cut into sections and mounted on glass slides.

The research focus for my laboratory was brain tumors and whether one could manipulate the immune system to restrict development and growth of tumors implanted in the brains of mice and now rats. We were trying to determine if there was effective immunotherapy against tumor growing in the central nervous system. In the second trial of a major monthlong experiment, all the control, sham-treated rats had died from progressive growth of their brain tumors, while only one of the treated group of rats with brain tumors was dead. This experiment, coupled with a previous trial, told us that with this new species and a different tumor, our treatment protocol still cured animals with brain tumors, and now could be tried against brain tumors in humans under experimental conditions approved by the FDA.

Excitement over our positive results was palpable. Scientific investigation is emotional, like betting on a horse race. Highs and lows run the full spectrum, from profound joy when studies yield important, consistent findings to intense dejection when results of experiments are negative, make no sense, or one is ruined because of a technical glitch. Published experimental results have to be reproducible not only by the original laboratory but also by any other laboratory using the same materials and methods. I had always found research to be very creative and a chance to expand my innate curiosity about biologic processes. As an engineer tied to more predictable tools and functions, Phil marvels at my willingness to try new methods, and is envious of the satisfaction I get with nothing more than simple exploration. But I was also well acquainted with drudgery—every exciting scientific breakthrough from my or any other laboratory is fueled by an incredible number of hours of tedious, repetitious, mind-numbing traverses over well-traveled roads.

Later I operated on an emergency basis on a patient with an almost totally blocked carotid artery, as "lab" days rarely can be devoted entirely to research. The patient had started having mini strokes twenty-four hours before. The neurologic occurrences, when he couldn't talk or move his right arm, would persist for a few minutes and then clear, leaving him perfectly intact. He had suffered two episodes that morning while eating breakfast, and after he dropped a cup of hot coffee, his worried wife convinced him he needed to see a doctor. She had brought him to the emergency room, where he continued to protest, "It's nothing serious—I'm O.K." An arteriogram demonstrated the expected occluding lesion at the bifurcation of his left carotid artery. At surgery, an ugly, ulcerated atherosclerotic plaque—its pathology reflected a history of smoking and a diet of too much red meat, eggs, and butter—was removed without difficulty. The resident working with me did a superb job, and the patient was neurologically intact after awakening from anesthesia. All of the work had gone well—it had been a good day.

Only one residual, nagging uncertainty remained—Philip. He was at our vacation home on the ocean with Xina, our Dalmatian, for company, maintaining his usual routine of leaving me with our two cats a few days each week so both of us could rekindle our spirits with a weekly spell of solitude. On a philosophical level he knew I would resign if Gerry was named chair, but I was not sure he was fully prepared for the reality of what I had done, and I had not yet told him of the dean's phone call. I finally phoned him that evening. When I told him about my resignation, his response made my heart sink lower than I thought possible: "Oh, my God, no." The abject despair was involuntary; he knew this was not easy for me.

"Is it effective today?" His sorrow and concern were relayed flawlessly by the miles of phone line.

"No. I thought I should finish out my term as Medical Faculty Senate chair. That isn't up until the first of September, so I made it effective then." Because the chair sits on the dean's Executive Committee, I wanted to retain the position and its access to confidential information for as long as possible, even though I would be a lame duck.

Phil grasped at what he saw as a glimmer of hope. "Good thinking—that gives you some time to change things."

As it happened, the Medical Faculty Senate convened the next day at a regularly scheduled meeting. The Senate has formal jurisdiction over admissions policy, curriculum, and student performance, but also serves as a forum to discuss any issues important to the medical school. The agenda for the meeting had been circulated the week before. I knew the major topic for discussion could be volatile. Some medical students had complained about something that had never been brought to the Senate before—sexual harassment. The Senate Steering Committee had already met with a small group of students and decided the concerns they articulated were valid and worthy of discussion by the faculty.

In 1991, sexual harassment, long an ingrained and traditional part of the medical world, was virtually never discussed, nor was it explicitly defined. I was aware Stanford had a history of sexual harassment, particularly in conjunction with my own department, but had chosen to ignore it because it was nebulous, secret, and did not seem particularly important to those who were in a position to stop it. It was a history I was about to discover in detail, the first link in a chain of episodes that finally opened my eyes to reality.

In 1986, while I was on sabbatical leave at the business school, a female lab technician working in neurosurgery had filed a sexual harassment complaint and then been terminated, ostensibly for "poor performance" but more probably because she had the temerity to file a further claim with the Equal Employment Opportunity Commission (EEOC) (which was eventually denied). She claimed she had been propositioned by Gerry. In addition, a married male neurosurgery resident had come to her house one evening armed with a six-pack of beer and an implicit invitation for sexual activity. A deeply religious person and a nondrinker, she declined both. Following the alleged episodes there was a decrement in her job performance, accompanied by unexplained crying spells. She was badly frightened and humiliated that her superiors considered her a woman with loose morals, and she never recovered her professional composure. I was aware that no action had been taken against either Gerry or the resident.

In 1988 Luann and Jolie had filed their grievances with the Human Resources Group, claiming they had been sexually harassed by Gerry. Although their complaints generated written affidavits within that office, the allegations were never investigated or made known to the medical school administration, because, the two women were informed, behavior they found offensive was subject to individual interpretation. They had also been told they could not expect their work environment to change. When they quit the Neurosurgery Department, they had been transferred to other jobs within the university.

Even though I had talked briefly with Luann and Jolie in 1988, I had no idea what had really happened or even how they had defined harassment. Before the Senate convened I now needed as much information as possible about the events. Just what did constitute sexual harassment, and why were the students so uptight about their learning environment?

Jolie and Luann were both still employed at Stanford, and a week before the Senate meeting (and before the dean's phone call about Gerry's appointment) they agreed to speak with me. Gerry was in the operating room, so we met in the neurosurgery clinic area and moved into one of the empty examining rooms, carefully closing the door. Luann and Jolie are good friends. They are high-energy women who were dedicated employees when they worked for neurosurgery. Both women were eager to share their stories.

They had received numerous thinly veiled invitations from Gerry for sexual activity—they were Hispanic, women, inferiors, and fair game. His frequent suggestive comments heard by everyone in the clinic area—such as "Let's you and me get it on, babe" and "Bet I could make you happy in bed, sweetheart"—were not really taken seriously, were met with hesitant giggling, but, at the same time, were demeaning and made the two women very uncomfortable. After all, he was a professor of neurosurgery and it was their job to help him. On occasion, they would "jokingly" be backed into corners, or spread-eagled against walls, where escape meant physically pushing the obstructing body while deflecting arms and hands. Close "hovering" was a common insult on days when Gerry was in clinic because he had frequent questions about his clinic schedule or a particular patient, and Jolie and Luann had the answers. The hovering posture included an arm draped around a feminine shoulder with a hand that would stray toward the breast. Both women became adept at rapidly turning their swivel chairs to confront Gerry face to face, decreasing the likelihood of being compromised by an unwelcome, intrusive hover.

I told them I was not surprised by their descriptions because I had seen some of it happen to them. But was this really "sexual harassment"? After all, Gerry was known to have a big mouth and doctors are very "touchy" people—examining people's bodies is what we do for our living. Were they confusing Gerry's actions with the innocent touching most of us in medicine are guilty of? Their situation was quite different from what went on in the surgical suite, where some surgeons had profound difficulty separating work from play. In the scrub sink area I had seen Gerry nibble on nurses' necks and ears or put his arms around their rib cages so their breasts and his arms were in contact. Not wanting to break their scrub cycle, either they would squirm to try to get away from him, which he enjoyed, or they did not seem particularly bothered. Some even appeared to invite attention from him.

Jolie answered without hesitation. "Dr. Conley—Fran— there's touching and then there's *touching*. I think both Luann and I know the difference." She looked straight at me and her voice was firm and confident.

I knew she was right; I also had no difficulty in distinguishing the difference. But I suddenly realized there was something that bothered me even more, something extraordinarily difficult to define. It was not only about touching and fondling—it was an attitude. In my department women had no value. I hate the term "sexism" because there's no "sexuality" per se in what I am talking about. I was not being pawed or handled in the clinic or office area—that only happened to me in the operating room or at departmental luncheons, away from conscious patients. But there was an implicit message in the neurosurgery office routine, and from Gerry's verbal comments, that I was inferior because I was a woman, and for no other reason. Gerry knew I could hold my own as a neurosurgeon, but somehow he did not see me as an equal. A number of women doctors have told me over the years that Gerry's attitude toward them suggested that if he was not sexually attracted to them, they simply did not exist. His usual and preferred method for diminishing women was to simply ignore them—they were entirely inconsequential.

All those years of toughing it out and not thinking about how I was being treated ended abruptly as my conversation with Luann and Jolie continued. All of us had been maligned, but in different ways. Gerry considered none of us to be serious professionals, and his "harassing" attitude and behavior had profoundly influenced all of our lives and careers. We warmly hugged each other goodbye, promising to stay in touch.

At the Senate meeting there was a standing-room-only crowd. I remember being very surprised by the turnout—usually we barely had a quorum. I just did not realize, even then, that the intense interest was emblematic of a deep-seated unrest that had spread not only within Stanford Medical School but also into many disciplines and workplaces across the entire country. Working women everywhere were demanding equal opportunity in work assignments, in advancement to managerial positions, equal pay for equal work, and an occupational environment of respect and dignity.

We spent the first fifteen minutes of the meeting approving minutes, and hearing obligatory reports from Dean Korn, the Dean of Admissions, and the standing committees of the Senate. I next established ground rules for the discussion that would follow, relying on notes and an earlier self-rehearsal. I told the crowd, "Two weeks ago the Senate Steering Committee heard about incidents of sexual harassment involving our medical students, as well as episodes of marked insensitivity when we consider that both genders are here learning to be doctors. The students feel they have a compromised educational environment, and the Steering Committee agrees with them. We also felt the

Senate was the most logical forum for discussing these issues, and I expect you, as representatives of your departments, to take the substance of today's discussion back to your constituents for further dialogue among yourselves."

I then directed my attention to the students who were sitting on the floor or standing at the back and sides of the horseshoe-shaped table where the senators were seated. "The Senate needs to hear about incidents, in as much detail as possible about what is going on. I will recognize any student who wishes to speak, but I don't want your name, or any names of involved parties you may talk about, so think in generalities before you ask for the floor. The minutes will reflect the substantive nature of your comments, but will contain no personal identification of you or others. I don't want this session to become a vendetta against a single person or a particular department. However, I do realize even if gender harassment problems exist only in isolated pockets, it still reflects on the total atmosphere of the school, and recently Dean Korn has gone on record, with written memos, that this type of misconduct will not be tolerated here."

I made no attempt to define what I meant by the term "sexual harassment," and Dean Korn did not offer his definition either. I had no idea why the dean had suddenly started writing numerous memos.

The meeting was opened for comments. A number of hands were raised, many tentatively, indicating both a desire and a reluctance to speak. I recognized one of the female students who had met with the Steering Committee two weeks before, figuring she would be daring enough to break the ice.

"I think I want to do surgery, and was told by one of the male surgery residents that I didn't have the right genes—to be a surgeon." She blushed a deep pink at her boldness, and ended by tittering, effectively reducing the strength of her words. But I was disturbed by her comment. Twenty-five years after I had fought to be a surgeon, female medical students were still hearing the same story I had. While I had actively encouraged women medical students who seemed well suited for a career in surgery to persist in their dreams, others were negating my support by telling them there was no place for them in that sacrosanct world of men.

Another woman spoke. "In one of my classes—our classes— the professor showed a slide of a blow-up doll—you know, the naked woman ones—and told us, 'Meet Angel, your new companion.' He was discussing respiratory physiology. I went to him after the class and said I thought his slide was offensive, and he told me *I* had a problem—*he* didn't." One of the faculty asked her how the slide had been connected to the subject of the lecture. "I really couldn't see any connection, sir."

Another female student added, "I'm not sure how to disguise this—this professor showed a printout of his wife's uterine contractions to the class and said, 'Of course, none of *you* will ever experience this.' And, I thought, can't he see who's in the audience? So much of the time our professors make us, as women, just simply disappear—we don't exist."

We heard more stories that day, most coming from women, most having to do with classroom sexism. One male student, intense, with a crew cut and thick glasses, said he felt, as a male, he had been discriminated against during his ob-gyn rotation. He had been prohibited from doing pelvic exams on certain patients and was not included in a doctor-patient encounter where sexual dysfunction had been discussed. He was convinced his learning experience in this discipline had not been equivalent to that of his female classmates. During a momentary lull, a professor of radiology, male, abruptly asked the student group, "Why did you men come to this meeting?"

"I'll be glad to tell you why—because we don't like what's happening to our female classmates." The speaker was obviously angry. "My girlfriend's been fighting off her goddamn chief resident for the past four weeks. He rubs up against her whenever he can, and pats her butt as a 'thank you' anytime she does a bit of scut work he's assigned to her. He's always got his hands on her. Last week she slapped him after he grabbed at her breast while she was working on a chart, and then he started tussling with her, locking her arms to keep her from slapping him again, and told her how cute she was when she got angry."

"What'd she do?"

"What do you mean, what'd she do? What *could* she do? He controls her. He's the one who does her evaluation, and she may need that evaluation for the residency she wants a year from now. If you guys think this is an isolated incident, think again—this guy's harassed every female student he's had on his service, and of course he gets away with it. They can't complain—a bad evaluation lives with you forever." There was a spattering of applause from the students for his bravery in speaking up.

The room was shocked into silence for a few moments. We absorbed the well-known, but never discussed notion that there was a potentially destructive component to the absolute power conferred by hierarchy. The students were trying to tell us we had spent our entire professional lives supporting a structure subject to abuse. It was one that now needed our help so that it might change.

Yet another male student raised his hand and asked about complaints two female medical students had filed against a professor in the medical school. I had heard only vague rumblings about the complaints, and knew none of the particulars. I was aware, though, there was considerable student unhappiness at the desultory and clandestine attempts by the administration either to resolve or to bury the two grievances. The student honored my request for no names, and I told him I could not provide the information he sought because I was not familiar with the case. In general, confidentiality rules precluded release of any information about a grievance against a faculty member until the case was investigated and settled. No other faculty spoke up either, although some, undoubtedly, were well acquainted with the facts.

The meeting was adjourned after I thanked the students for their participation. I also told them the meeting would not be the end to faculty action about these issues of pervasive sexism and sexual harassment at their medical school.

What I did not tell them was that I had resigned two days before, although the disclosure would have added a dramatic conclusion. I needed time to sort out my own conflicting thoughts and emotions. Where did my life fit into the picture that had just been painted? Did my concerns about Gerry, which were very real to me, but as yet inadequately synthesized and lacking cohesion, parallel those of the student group? As I drove home that evening I was left with a confused sense of déjà vu from my days as a medical student in the 1960s, coupled with the sober realization that cultural change within an institution was not dependent on the passage of time alone. Despite a class composition of 40 percent women, in 1991 the educational environment was not significantly different from the one I had experienced thirty years before, and if left unchanged, would continue to have a negative impact on the careers of these young women. The women were still expected to conform to male standards of behavior and, without questioning it, humbly accept the fact that they will never be perceived to be "as good as" their male compatriots.

The Senate meeting was the final blow. With sudden crisp clarity I realized I had been, and still was, a target of "sexual harassment" (a most inadequate label) and that my work world was one of blatant gender discrimination. Many actions by some of my male colleagues communicated total disrespect for me and my career, and devalued my competence and performance, in terms of both my past accomplishments and my future potential.

Therefore, I had some tough questions to answer for myself. Why had I been so blind? If not blind, exactly, just willing to look the other way? Like most women, I hate confrontation. Up to 1991 my professional career had progressed because I was willing to be a "good sport" and accept harassment, rather than challenge or question it and risk alienation, dismissal, or not being promoted. Instead, I chose to join the existing system, and had used that system, created by and for men, very well. Female friends were virtually absent from my life, I had only a couple of much younger professional female peers in surgery at Stanford, and I had never learned to respect women. So, in a time-honored way, I yearned for and actively sought approval from men, and defined myself within and by that male approval. I had made my peer group of surgical faculty my friends as well as my professional colleagues. Maintaining their friendship had been essential for my continued career development and academic survival. I certainly had not wanted any of them to be uncomfortable when I was around just because I was a "girl." Daily we shared a vocabulary of technical language as well as liberal use of four-letter words. My language was just as rotten as theirs. Episodes of inappropriate behavior had not diminished my fondness for them as a collective group. I was accustomed to games played to determine whether, and how far, I would cross a given line. I was well acquainted with raucous laughter erupting at my expense over jokes, nuances, antics, guesses about how good I was in bed. One survived in this masculine world by being one of the boys, and for all intents and purposes I had become one of them. Only I received much more physical attention, having legs that were stroked, a neck that was caressed, breasts that were a topic of conversation as to their size and shape. Frequently offended, I dared not offend, for fear of banishment from the only professional camaraderie I had ever known. Not wanting to lose my quasi membership in the surgeons' club, I had never done anything to stop behavior that was repulsive to me and ultimately damaging to my self-respect and dignity. Instead I had developed a fine art of repartee. I, too, could be insulting, using our dirty language to turn their faces red. Deflecting put-downs with humor, I earned the reputation of being able to fend for myself, and had developed tremendous pride in having that ability.

Inherently, I knew sexist behavior was wrong, but thought I was above it and had been able to keep it from hurting *my* career. Now, after the Senate meeting, I realized I might well have damaged the professional lives of others, because my own inaction, over the years, was as responsible as any other factor for perpetuating the sexist climate medical students found abhorrent and were now fighting.

And even though I was well educated about the political process that governed the medical school and had a position of power within the faculty, as well as great visibility, none of this had been, or was, enough to protect me. In fact, no woman in the medical arena had adequate protection. The occasional, carefully selected woman is permitted to accrue power, but, in reality, it is only decorative. She is never expected to use it. I had been a safe choice because I had genuinely and wholeheartedly bought into the system and ostensibly was a controllable part of it. Finally, I now understood that the essential functions of our medical world depended on women's willingness to capitulate to masculinity without asking questions, without fighting injustice, with complete servility, because maleness is the purest and most highly revered form of power in our profession.

I was overwhelmed by a profound sense of guilt. My resignation would not change anything. Unless there was a major shift in the way the medical world taught and assimilated its physicians, another generation of women doctors would endure the same abusive conditions I had encountered, believing, as I had, that it was a requirement for membership in the club. For some, the experience of being treated as inferior beings during their medical training would alter them forever, and envelop them with a crippling inferiority complex of self-doubt—a physician condemned to a lifetime of daily self-assessment about her own professional competence. Every morning, as they shave, my male colleagues tell their reflected images, "I'm the greatest." By contrast, my morning reflection, as I apply makeup, is asked whether I am good enough to meet the challenges of that day. It was counterproductive for more women doctors to relive my years of self-doubt. The system had to change so they could build their careers based on personal strength and self-confidence.

5 The next day, Saturday, I helped Phil with some yard work. It was a symbolic effort. For the best years of my life I had devoted weekends to reading and writing research papers and grant applications. Now I was acknowledging I had extra time. Phil's bush and tree trimming progressively liberated our view down the hill across the flatland to the bay, over to the East Bay hills dominated by Mount Diablo. As I raked the fresh, green aromatic branches into piles on the concrete patio, I thought about my resignation and the Senate meeting of the previous afternoon. Was a silent exit into the sunset all there was? Was I being fair to all those who had helped me develop a unique career? Was I cheating Phil, who had sacrificed so much? And what about the students, the nurses on our ward, Luann and Jolie, and all the others? Gerry had reached the pinnacle of academic neurosurgery. His appointment validated his behavior and ensured that his sexist ideology would be copied by the next generation of male neurosurgeons eager for success—to be just like him. The students had requested a culture change. Gerry's appointment was antithetical to their plea.

By the time the yard work was finished, I had decided to write an opinion piece, to let friends know why I was leaving, and to share with the world a glimpse of what was happening at Stanford. I was willing to go, but not without explanation. I finished writing the article that weekend.

On Tuesday morning, after doing a back operation at the VA to remove a ruptured lumbar disk, I called a friend, Marlys Labelle, in the Communications Department at Stanford, and asked if she had time to meet with me. It had been almost a week, and still there had been no announcement from Dean Korn about either Gerry's promotion to chair or my resigning from the faculty. He had not even formally acknowledged my resignation with a written memo. In fact, there had been absolutely no contact. I half expected him to call and ask to meet with me before he accepted it, to talk about Gerry, to discuss in greater detail my reasons for resigning and the repercussions of the resignation for both of us. Had he done so, the large-scale crisis that enveloped him, the school, and me might have been averted.

I had known Professor Labelle for years. She is a superb journalist with good contacts in the print media. I told Marlys I hoped my article would appear as an opinion piece with my byline, and would she mind editing it? She quickly scanned what I had written, then read it a second time, slowly and critically, making changes to smooth the syntax. When finished, she pushed her glasses onto the top of her head, leaned back in her chair, and asked if I would not rather wait a couple of weeks before I tried to publish it. Perhaps instinctively Marlys recognized the volatility of the subject, but she now contends she anticipated only a minor impact. Waiting was out of the question. In two weeks the students would be gone for the summer vacation, and I wanted them to know at least one faculty member had responded to the concerns they had brought to the Senate.

In the end, Marlys told me she thought the piece was publishable and gave me the names and addresses of the editors of six editorial pages, including four in the Bay Area. I sent the final version to the chosen newspapers:

I have resigned my position as a full tenured professor of a surgical specialty at a prominent U.S. medical school. Hard work over the past 23 years got me to the position I no longer hold and most observers, knowing of my successes, would have said, "You had it all." And I did—except for personal dignity.

Those who administer my work environment at the present time have never been able to accept me as an equal person. Not because I lack professional competence, but because I use a different bathroom. I am minus the appropriate gender identification that permits full membership in the club.

Most medical school classes today across the United States are composed of at least 35 percent women; in many the percentage is higher. Last week at my institution, medical students, both men and women, in approximately equal and impressive numbers, attended a meeting of the Faculty Senate to share with elected faculty representatives concerns over their work and study environment.

Even today, faculty are using slides of *Playboy* centerfolds to "spice up" lectures; sexist comments are frequent and those who are offended are told to be "less sensitive." Unsolicited touching and fondling occur between house staff and students, with the latter having little recourse to object. To complain might affect a performance evaluation. The subsequent ramifications could damage career paths and may extend well into the future.

The Faculty Senate meeting addressed the need to define objectionable behavior among our academic medical community. Students pleaded for change in the present environment to one where one gender can respect the other, assuring equality of learning and training opportunities for all.

It is probably true that, at least in the past, medicine has tended to attract men most comfortable in a society where males dominate subservient females. This society of men is most developed in surgery, where there are defined hierarchical parameters.

In general, surgery has been served well by a rigid structure of discipline that ensures most encounters between surgeon and patient are a success of life over death. The system is threatened, however, when a woman becomes a surgeon and long-standing rules establishing hierarchy of men over women no longer apply.

A few summers ago I invited a friend who is a professor of organizational behavior to examine power relationships in an operating-room environment. My contention was that I used power and my position as the surgeon quite differently from my male counterparts. He found female surgeons tend to manage their operating rooms with a team approach; male surgeons remain "captains of the ship." Of significance, both methods can provide good patient outcome.

When working with surgeons who are women, the nursing staff (predominantly women but also a few men) stated they felt more valued as fellow professionals—male surgeons were far less inclined to thank or praise their team at the successful completion of a case. Anger on the part of a male surgeon led to increased subservience by the nursing staff; humor was used much more frequently by women surgeons to achieve the same goal. An operating room is a very confined unit and women have been successful in adapting this environment to their special managerial styles.

Unfortunately, there is the world in academic medicine

outside of the operating theater—one composed of clinics, teaching, insurance forms, lawyers, research, administration, and politics. The administrative structure of American medicine today remains dominated by men, many of whom were raised by doting parents who considered them very special and superior beings. Even in my wonderful, egalitarian, liberal, academic family my brother was rewarded with a life insurance policy for the dubious distinction of reaching the age of 16; for like achievement my sisters and I were given sewing machines.

Surgical training certainly reinforces the concept of male superiority, and is sufficiently focused and demanding that, for some men, personality growth is truncated, leaving them in a time warp of persistent delusions about male and/or personal superiority. Such a person lacks the capacity to respond and adjust to societal changes. The danger for the future of medicine (and, I suspect, business and law) comes when one of these stunted individuals, who may be very gifted technically as physician, lawyer, or businessman, is assigned a position with authority over the professional lives of others.

In the distant past, when I was the only woman training in surgery at my institution, a fellow resident surgeon (married, as was I) used to delight in asking me to go to bed with him. The invitation was offered a number of times, always in jest and always in the company of others—always men. The purpose? Perhaps he was playing a game of "mine is bigger than yours" but I doubt it. In truth, I believe that this surgeon felt that women were created to feed him, clean up after him, and provide sexual gratification. Period. He had not even considered that I was his equal as a person, despite very similar educational backgrounds, intellect, and professional ability. His male superiority complex robbed him of any ability to accept me as a peer—the only way he could relate at all was to reduce our relationship to a level where there were clearly defined roles for a man and a woman.

In my letter of resignation, I described my work environment of the past 24 months as "hostile." Triggering the resignation was a decision that precipitously turned what I had hoped to be a temporary situation into a permanent one with regard to departmental leadership. Now at age 50 and looking ahead to the next 10 to 15 years of my career, I decided I didn't need to continue hearing myself described as "difficult."

As a fellow faculty member, I felt I had the right to express an honest difference of opinion but found any deviation on my part from the majority view often was announced prominently as a manifestation of either PMS syndrome or being "on the rag." I find myself unwilling to be called "hon" or "honey" with the same degree of sweet condescension used by this department for all women— nurses, secretaries, administrative assistants, female medical students.

Will anything be gained by my leaving a truly fine academic position? Many will view the move as a defeat, a failure, a lack of toughness, a loss of will to survive in a dog-eat-dog world. I hope that the answer is "yes"; that the future encompasses the rebuilding of my self-esteem and personal dignity.

However, I have no illusions that my leaving will benefit the present classes of medical students who seek institutional change. Instead, I leave in place a validated legacy of sexism, a role model for all men, that women are, indeed, inferior and expected to remain so.

A week and a day after I had hand-delivered my resignation notice, and two days after copies of the opinion piece had been mailed, Dean Korn dictated a "personal and confidential" memo to me, the subject of which was "Notice of Resignation." Although I realized my resignation was not the only item on the dean's agenda, I could not imagine why it had taken him so long to acknowledge it. Possibly he did not believe I was serious and was waiting for me to regain my senses and crawl back, begging his forgiveness. At the very least I believe he should have been concerned about losing one of his few female tenured full professors. Despite considerable rhetoric, repeated year after year, about the desirability of increasing the number of women faculty at the level of full professor, the words remain just words; the few of us with the rank remain a scarce commodity in academic medicine.

In his memo to me, dated May 31, the dean first detailed the school's financial woes and then wrote, ". . . you have left me with no alternative but to accept it [the resignation]. . . . I understand you and Gerry have had a long-standing interpersonal difficulty, and I genuinely regret that, also. I agree with you that no one should be forced to live their lives in misery. . . . Finally, I wish you well in whatever future endeavor you choose to pursue." His letter had been copied to President Donald Kennedy.

Gerry also dictated a short, perfunctory letter to me the same day. I had not told him about resigning. The dates on the two letters were the same, leading me to believe the two men had talked sometime that Friday. Unlike the dean, Gerry did not delay in acknowledging my action. Then he left for a short vacation. His letter was more formal and much briefer:

Dear Dr. Conley:

It is with great sadness that I accept your resignation. I regret that you have elected to resign rather than remain on the faculty and help us develop a truly outstanding neurosurgery program. I know that I speak for all of our Depart-

ment when I say that we will miss your expertise and that
we wish you the best of luck in all of your endeavors.

Yours sincerely,
Gerald D. Silverberg, M.D.
Professor and Acting Chairman
Department of Neurosurgery

It was signed with an impersonal full signature. He had won. I had lost.

Neither Gerry nor the dean addressed my unusual move of resigning a tenured full professorship to register objection over a choice for executive leadership. Between the lines, I read a sense of relief and some eagerness to help implement my departure as expeditiously and quietly as possible. Despite Gerry's protests of "sadness," my departure was freeing up a faculty slot. The dissident was leaving, and he could now recruit a young neurosurgeon of his choice.

Late Friday afternoon I was sitting in my office reviewing a legal case, waiting for a phone call from Stanford telling me the resident staff was ready to make evening rounds. I was the on-call staff neurosurgeon for the weekend and had to cover both VA and Stanford hospitals. But when the phone rang, it was not the chief resident. A Michael McCabe from the *San Francisco Chronicle* told me his op-ed editor had just handed him my piece and had asked that he find out what was really happening. The call was unexpected. I had thought my article would just be published, no questions asked, and had not considered the possibility there would be any inquiry about what I had written. I was just trying to share what was happening in neurosurgery with the rest of the world—what more did he want? I told McCabe what I had written was true and that I was willing to talk to him about it.

But McCabe wanted to know the identity of the person I had

challenged. He was after a sensational me-versus-him story. Without mentioning Gerry by name, I told him "this person" was but one of many with ingrained sexist beliefs, that most abuse toward women in the medical field was verbal, subtle, ubiquitous, and probably unconscious. It was the additive nature of daily slights, confirming for all women our second-class citizenship on a regular basis, that was most offensive, robbing us of self-esteem, dignity, and respect. How can any patient take me seriously, I said, when I'm called "honey" by the department chair? When McCabe asked, I acknowledged that there was a touchy-feely quality to many personal contacts that probably did not belong in a professional environment. I also said that the only way our culture would change was through more enlightened leadership. My resignation was in protest over an executive choice the dean had made, where the behavior I described would be validated and perpetuated for another generation.

I inquired whether he planned to publish my opinion piece. He answered it was not his decision, that he was just a reporter and his editor thought there might be a story. He abruptly told me he had a deadline to meet and thanked me for my time. I hung up the phone and took a deep breath. How was I to know I had just lost control of my world?

That night, sleep was strangely elusive. By 5:30 a.m. I was wide awake. Our morning newspaper had already been delivered. When I picked up the *Chronicle*, I was stunned by a front-page article and headline: "Stanford Brain Surgeon Quits Over 'Sex Harassment.'" In his short, sensational piece, Michael McCabe wrote glibly of "years of sexual harassment" and recounted incidents of fondling and groping. Although I do not remember having said it, a quote attributed to me read, "There is a very fine line between wanting to 'belong' and wanting to make an issue of it. I have decided to make an issue of it." He had also managed to reach the dean, who was quoted as saying, "I am not exactly sure what motivated her to do this, although I do know she has had a difficult interpersonal relationship with a colleague." Korn had refused to comment on the charges of "sexual harassment." McCabe finished his article with a quote from Dr. Margaret Billingham, professor of pathology at Stanford and a good friend of mine. "When a woman becomes a senior member of faculty, particularly in surgery, men perceive her as a threat. It's like women in the Army. Surgery is supposed to be men's business" (*San Francisco Chronicle*, June 1, 1991). My editorial had not been published.

That morning I had to join the residents for rounds. Reluctantly, I drove down the hill to the hospital, very uneasy about meeting them. To my knowledge, they were still unaware I had resigned. I wished I could disappear for a while and let the volatile story self-destruct. I walked down the wide hospital corridor feeling totally conspicuous, as if everyone I passed had read the morning *Chronicle*, knew who I was, and was staring at me. Two residents and two interns waited for me in the radiology reading room. None of them had seen the morning paper. Hesitantly, I told them about the front-page article and its sensational headline, continuing, "It's true I've resigned as professor of neurosurgery, effective the first of September, but really not over what *I* would call 'sexual harassment.' I quit because of the way Gerry treats me, and the way he regards all women as inferior, and because he's always belittling someone. I'm embarrassed by his behavior and I don't want to be a part of that department where he's chair." I asked whether they knew he was now the permanent chair of the department. They remained silent and all solemnly nodded "yes."

"I really want to apologize to you for the sensationalism. I did write an editorial, but the papers have added their own unfortunate slant. I didn't name Gerry or the department, or even the school in what I wrote, but around here, everyone will know, and I'm sure you'll have to answer some questions. I'm sorry for making your lives more difficult." My eyes filled with tears as the awkward silence continued.

Finally the chief resident cleared his throat and said he was sorry I would be leaving.

My voice broke as I thanked him, then said, "Let's roll." I quickly brushed the tears from my eyes as we left the room to begin morning rounds.

The *Chronicle* story on "rampant sexism" at the Stanford Medical School ran on the AP wire, and many Sunday papers across the country chose to run it. I had sent my opinion piece to the *San Jose Mercury News* and the *Peninsula Times Tribune*, and both used material taken from it to augment the wire release. The Sunday *San Francisco Examiner* headlined its story: "New Stanford Furor: Med School Sexism," then below, in slightly smaller print: "Surgeon resigns, saying she's seen too much abuse." The story ended with a quote from Dean Korn: " 'I don't doubt that there are members of the medical profession who might be sexist or biased in one way or another, that they trade jokes and expressions that persons who don't belong to the white-male majority might find offensive.' But that falls short of harassment, he said, expressing concern about infringing on the rights of free speech. Harassment, said Korn, would not be tolerated. 'If cases are brought to us we will deal with them vigorously and effectively' " (*San Francisco Examiner*, June 2, 1991).

I was still uncertain how Dean Korn himself defined "harassment," but thought I now understood why he had not been particularly interested when I told him about my problems with Gerry. He believed Gerry's free speech rights were inviolate, and that abusive gender-based verbalization neither constituted "sexual harassment" nor precluded appointment to executive leadership.

Phil returned from our ocean house late Saturday afternoon. He had already seen McCabe's article but, along with me, wondered why it appeared in isolation from the opinion piece I had written. He has a healthy distrust of the media, but surprised me by expressing pleasure in his belief that writing the editorial had generated some effect. We spent Sunday answering numerous supportive phone calls from friends across the country.

After the weekend of phone calls the dog and I ran an extra mile Monday morning, and I enjoyed a leisurely morning cup of coffee. The day was entirely free, as my scheduled all-day case to remove a difficult brain tumor had been canceled by the attending anesthesiologist. Along with my usual outfit of slacks and running shoes I chose to wear a simple pink T-shirt depicting a fat white cat on the front accompanied by the wording "Owner of the world's cutest cat." I was totally unprepared for what was happening at the office.

When my secretary, Rita Ulheim, arrived at eight, the phone was ringing and the voice mail was full. When I walked in forty-five minutes later, the phone was still ringing and the voice mail had not been cleared. Nancy, the pleasant, almost motherly public relations person for the VA, met me as I came up the stairs to the back entrance into the surgical suite. "At least three television stations will be here at ten for an interview. Hope you don't mind. I'll have them set up in the conference room."

"What . . . ?" I answered.

Nancy and I walked the few steps from the door to Rita's desk, and Rita looked up from the phone at me and said, "I phoned you at home to warn you, and Phil said you'd just left."

I was appalled. I had hoped the weekend story would have made its little splash and then drowned. I never expected the VA to be invaded, and certainly had not anticipated this intensity of interest in Michael McCabe's sleazy story. I had been incredibly naive. McCabe himself had interpreted the incidents recounted in the opinion piece as "sexual harassment," pure and simple. By labeling them as such, he ignited a wildfire of interest about the inside workings of the medical school and how women were treated there. I could have refused to meet with the media and perhaps stopped the story right then. But I was intrigued by what they found so fascinating about my world. The only stories about "sexual harassment" that had come to my attention were incidents where sexual favors were demanded and received in exchange for job promotions, or a woman had been physically assaulted by her boss while at work. The story I had to tell was very tame by comparison.

Most of the surgical suite at the VA is an open work area, surrounded at its perimeter by individual doctors' offices. So everyone witnessed the arrival of television crews and their excessive paraphernalia from the three Bay Area networks. I had escaped to my office and was answering phone calls when Nancy and one of the TV people came to the door to tell me they were ready. Suddenly I remembered the silly T-shirt. I pulled my white lab coat off its hanger and put it on, buttoning it closed, almost hiding the stupid cat. It's too bad if television doesn't like the white color, I thought. I also hoped the cameras would stay away from my running shoes.

The three reporters, two women and one man, were elegantly dressed. As I greeted them, I was grateful I had chosen a career where fashionable dress was not expected on a daily basis. For much of my workweek I wear scrub greens or blues, covered, when necessary, by a white lab coat with my name embroidered above the left breast pocket. It is a simple, but imposing uniform. The standard hospital scrub outfits are baggy, reversible, laundered by the institution, and infinitely comfortable—similar to wearing sturdy pajamas all day long.

The television newspeople asked me to talk about the medical school and the issues that had brought them to my office. I told them, "The dean has gone on record saying this medical school will provide an educational experience for its students that is egalitarian and where students have the opportunity to develop themselves to their maximum potential regardless of gender, race, or sexual orientation. There's good reason to believe we haven't achieved that goal yet, but according to the dean, the commitment remains. I believe a grievous error was made a little more than a week ago in one of his choices for executive leadership. The dean appointed a person as the chair of my Department of

Neurosurgery who, in my opinion, is the epitome of a sexist pig."

I instantly regretted my language, but continued, "This person has never been able to accept me as a neurosurgeon, not because I'm not capable, but because I'm a woman. I've put up with his demeaning actions and words for twenty-five years and have watched him belittle other women, notably nursing staff and secretaries. All of us are his 'honeys.' Well, you know something? We aren't. If anyone is, his wife's his 'honey.' "

One of the reporters asked if I had wanted the job—they had heard this whole publicity stunt was just a sour grapes reaction on my part. I told them the search committee had never seen my résumé. I was an official "noncandidate."

I should have expected the next question: "What's his name?" With only a slight pause of surprise, I answered, "I'm not here to provide names; the problem is a generic one, and this person isn't the only colleague of mine who's guilty of this type of behavior."

"Dr. Conley, what types of behavior are you talking about?"

"I'm sorry, but this isn't a story about rape, plunder, and pillage, as the newspaper coverage would have you believe and what you want to hear. Yes, inappropriate touching and fondling are a part of my work world, but the larger issue is much more subtle, and has to do with being measured not by one's abilities but by one's gender or skin color. And the types of behavior that elicit a feeling of second-class citizenship for women and minorities are very difficult to delineate. This isn't a problem that can be defined in black and white—it's gray, a whole spectrum of gray." I stopped.

"Dr. Conley, there's no story in gray." One of the women reporters said this without a smile and was absolutely serious.

I thought to myself, "This is what's wrong with the media in this country," but said to her, "I think there is a story, and I think it's an important one, one that truly will dictate how we as a country incorporate diversity into our workforce. What I'm talking about isn't unique to this medical school, or even to medicine. In law women don't get partnerships, in business they never rise above middle management; women in political office are as rare as a female neurosurgeon. And your profession hasn't been particularly kind to women. We hear a few more women on radio and now see a few more on television, but so frequently it isn't your talent that keeps your jobs for you, it's your looks. A few gray hairs and wrinkles and you're out. Do you think any television producer would use a woman on-camera who had aged like Mike Wallace or Morley Safer? I think you face job pressures that men in your profession, by and large, don't—let me know if I'm wrong. And where are the women in production and management in media enterprises? You have to realize, at the medical school where we're teaching doctors to care for you—the patient—the culture is such that women as patients get a raw deal too. As they go through a training program, young doctors adopt the thinking and prejudices of their professors—these are the people they revere, the ones they want to be like someday. To align themselves with their professors' mental attitudes, male students also gradually come to believe women can't really think, are like children, and they begin treating them as such. They never see women patients as equal partners in health care, where decisions are made about their medical needs—they dictate to them, and fully expect women to accept whatever they say and recommend, without question. In fact, many male surgeons I know accept questions from their male patients as being part of their job, but are truly affronted when a female patient dares question their advice, or has the audacity to reject a surgical procedure, or even ask for a second opinion. The medical sexist culture influences many more lives than just those of women doctors."

There was momentary silence. Then the male reporter said the group needed something more concrete for their viewers and began asking about the examples covered in the newspaper article.

For the next five minutes I tried to explain how gender-specific comments and gestures affected my ability to function as a neurosurgeon, and told them why I had not felt compelled to speak out earlier, how I tried to warn the administration about "this person," and refused to speculate on what I would do with my life come the first of September. The session ended cordially, although I felt the media group was vaguely dissatisfied.

As the television crews prepared to leave, Rita told me there were two photographers waiting: one from *The New York Times*, the other from a newspaper syndicate—this whole thing was rapidly becoming larger than life.

Despite a huge backup of unanswered phone calls, and requests for my time, at noon I closed my office door, asked Rita not to disturb me, and wrote a note to the dean on my computer, figuring he deserved some explanation for the unprogrammed disruption to his day. I apologized for the media sensationalism but not for having raised the issue of ubiquitous sexism at the medical school. I acknowledged he might have some difficulty understanding the hostility of my work environment, because I doubted he himself had ever endured a similar one, where demeaning verbalizations were an accepted mode of communication. My memo ended, "Promoting Gerry to department chair validates his pervasive sexist attitudes and because he has been successful in his career he will serve as a role model for the next generation of male surgeons, thus reinventing and perpetuating the time warp of male dominant, female subservient roles. If we are to provide an environment for learning, study, and training for the next generation of physicians where all can be considered equal peers, and can learn to respect not only themselves but others, regardless of differences, then Gerry's appointment is a true step in the wrong direction."

I enclosed a copy of my unpublished opinion piece. I wanted Korn to know that what I had written was not that sensational or newsworthy, that it was just a description of my professional life, which he already knew about.

I felt better for having written the letter, because the exercise clearly defined the issues as I saw them. I was not at all convinced, however, that Dean Korn would be similarly enlightened, and subliminally was aware that many others, also, would not understand. This was not a popular cause. Phil's experience told me I was right.

At noontime he often jogged with an assorted group of men and women, some from Stanford, some from surrounding high-tech companies, of variable age and running talent. In addition to a physical workout, these meetings served as a social outlet for Phil, one where he could gossip and joke with others without significantly intertwining his life with theirs. That Monday he heard a number of unsolicited opinions, some of which forced a redefinition of his concept of "friend." True friends assumed I had done something I felt had to be done, no questions asked—genuine concern and offers to help were extended. From others, soon to be nonfriends, Phil heard hypotheses of an adulterous romance gone awry, unrequited professional ambition, bitchy vindictiveness aimed at further tarnishing Stanford's public image, a sudden, unacceptable hook to the caboose of feminism.

I spent the rest of that mad, topsy-turvy Monday answering requests for interviews, doing a few interviews, posing for more photographs, answering long-distance phone calls, and talking with friends from the university. I also received a number of un-expected comforting calls from women who wanted to share stories with me about their interactions with Gerry. Although I had not named him, our community knew exactly who it was I had challenged. One of the early helpful calls I received was from Professor Lois Sweet, one of two female chairs at the medical school. Because I already knew plenty about Gerry's behavior and had no need to hear more, I asked her to act as a clearinghouse for information, especially about Gerry, from people who felt like sharing. Graciously she agreed to have these phone calls trans-ferred to her office. Another good friend, Professor Corinne Spitz, a tenured full professor in neurobiology, called from the airport to express dismay, and then said she, too, very probably would soon be leaving Stanford. I was astonished; Corinne is a superstar with an international scientific reputation. She had developed her illustrious career at Stanford, and her continued presence on the faculty attracted the very best doctoral candidates and postdoctoral fellows. Dean Korn could not afford to lose her without having his own reputation suffer.

When David Korn came to work on Monday, he faced the same degree, or more, of media attention that I did. His public relations advisors had arranged a press conference for the afternoon in order to satisfy the media appetite with a single feeding. By the time of the gathering, a press release had been written, and abbreviated segments of his response, carried by radio and television that evening, did not differ substantially from this written text. A few days later, a picture taken at the press conference was printed on the front page of the *Campus Report*, a weekly publication for the Stanford community. In it Dean Korn is seated behind a bouquet of microphones flanked by his two grim-faced senior associate deans. The audience was so large it spilled out the exit door. The atmosphere was not joyous. An unusual, and unexpected, number of interested people from the medical community were in attendance.

In the press release the dean reviewed the circumstances leading to my resignation, but failed to mention a "hostile environment," stating only that I had been "unhappy with his decision." He acknowledged I was an important role model but also mentioned that, because I had received a degree from the business school, I had been contemplating a change in my professional career—thus giving the media a motive for my actions. Korn stated, "Accordingly, I have written many letters of reference on Professor Conley's behalf with respect to open positions in academic health centers. . . . I have prepared my reference letters with enthusiasm and sincerity. I shall continue to wish her well in her quest."

Next the press release moved abruptly to consideration of the Medical Faculty Senate meeting. "A few of the students presented anecdotes of what seemed to me to be clearly instances of inappropriate conduct, but in the main, the majority of the discussion dealt with a variety of issues, largely in the areas of gender insensitivity, that were clearly stated to involve both sexes. Stanford University has had for a number of years a clear policy about sexual harassment. I wish to state clearly for the record that the school of medicine does not and will not tolerate inappropriate sexual behaviors or actions, for they degrade the learning and working environment of the institution. Any such behaviors that are brought to the attention of the dean's office will be dealt with vigorously, fairly, and effectively." However, nowhere in the release did Dean Korn give his operational definition of sexual harassment. He added, "In this respect, it is important to state that to the best of my knowledge, Professor Conley has never brought a specific complaint of sexual misbehavior or harassment to the attention of any administrative officer of the school of medicine or the university."

He ended with a soothing mea culpa. "We still have much work to do in changing attitudes, beliefs, and behaviors within our profession, to eliminate bigotry and bias and to make the medical profession more hospitable and nurturing to its women and ethnic minority members. Historically the profession has been dominated by white males, and insensitivity and intolerance doubtless continue among us. The culture of the profession will change, but equally inevitably, that change will only occur by evolution over a period of time."

In his question-and-answer session with media representatives, Dean Korn revealed Professor Gerald Silverberg was the chair-elect I had refused to identify. He also said, in response to reporters' queries, "I would love Dr. Conley to stay. I don't think losing Frances Conley is good for the community."

Korn correctly was attempting to keep the situation from escalating, but I felt quite defensive about how he had couched some of his comments. For example, Korn recognized little or no connection between my resignation and sexism, and negated my right to even raise the possibility because I had never brought a specific complaint of "sexual harassment" to his attention. He trivialized, then dismissed, the concerns of the students. I freely admit he had written an embarrassingly large number of letters of recommendation for me, especially after 1989 when we had more frequent contact because I chaired the Senate. It was more than a little bizarre, and I had no idea then why he felt compelled to write them. These letters were unsolicited by me, and he had not inquired about my interest in any of the jobs before writing. I lacked the requisite qualifications in upper-level academic administration for 99 percent of the jobs which he identified and for which had submitted my name. I had written letters, equal in number to his, requesting my name be withdrawn from any consideration. I assumed the letters had been written in good faith, and was mildly flattered that he had such confidence in me, but wish the dean had attempted to match my abilities with the requirements for each particular job before wasting my time, his time, and the time of the inquiring institution.

Reporters who came to the VA late Monday afternoon told me about medical students placing a large paper banner in the medical school courtyard, proclaiming "Bravo, Dr. Conley," and smaller placards, with the same message, being taped onto campus directory maps which are strategically located on all streets leading to the center. A huge beautiful bouquet of mixed flowers arrived from the medical center operating room nurses. The small accompanying card read simply, "Thanks."

Overnight, because of the power of the media, I became something I was not. I knew next to nothing about the feminist movement, feminist causes, or even what it meant to be labeled a "feminist." While I have always believed in equality of opportunity for women and minorities, I had never been a militant constituent of any organized cause. I supported women's groups on campus, but had taken no active role in their management, and belonged to no national women's organizations except for Women in Neurosurgery, which had just been organized—again, without input from me. I was the least likely of candidates to lead this particular crusade with its huge following. All I had done was resign an academic position because my career was finished anyway. For my own selfish survival, I had seen no alternative to what I had done.

I stopped at Stanford on my way home from the VA, figuring it was late enough to pick up my mail without encountering any of the staff. I was amazed at the volume of cards, short notes, and letters I found. Most were local, many from friends and colleagues at the university—brief expressions of "Congratulations," "Thank you," "Bravo," "I'm so sorry," "How can I help?" Others were longer, already prognosticating the future where I would wear the mantle for "every woman," a costume with a very poor fit. At the bottom of the pile was a computer-generated message on a single sheet of paper that read, "Good for you!!! Cheers to you, Dr. Conley for your sacrifice and courage!" In handwriting on the diagonal at the bottom right corner was, "You have no idea what you have tapped into! A Stanford employee."

▾6▾ An edited version of my opinion piece was finally published on the editorial page of the *San Francisco Chronicle* on Tuesday morning, June 4, followed by a heavily edited version of David Korn's press release from the previous day. Both the *Peninsula Times Tribune* and the *San Jose Mercury News* published my entire piece that evening.

In rereading the article, I found it difficult to understand how it had catalyzed what was becoming a national furor. While the words "sexist" and "sexism" are used in it, there is no mention of "sexual harassment." The environment depicted probably was not even unique to Stanford University School of Medicine. But the thought that women were being mistreated in any way by doctors—those gracious, caring professionals who are entrusted with our most intimate confidences—was ammunition enough to ignite a firestorm of concern. Was there a carefully hidden, secret part of the medical profession—a dark world of tarnished ethics and abuse of power? Thomas C. Benet, chief editorial writer for the *San Francisco Chronicle*, wrote a short letter thanking me for sending the article, stating he thought the "piece was well-written, cogent and very much to the point."

I phoned Benet and, with restraint, thanked him for his kind words. What I really wanted to do was scream at him. He and McCabe had it all wrong. The label "sexual harassment" was too convenient, too encompassing, too sensational, too sleazy, too ill defined. It evoked an eye-winking response from some men, disbelief from others, and a frequent reaction of "Oh well, *you* must have done something to lead him on." It smacked of degeneracy, reduced the problem to a personal level, and voided the seriousness of my overarching concerns about leadership and the future of medicine. The issue for most professional women was not about being sexually coerced or abused—our concern was over being trivialized solely on account of our gender, and the repercussions of that trivialization on our subsequent careers. Yet for want of a better term, "sexual harassment" was what I was stuck with, thanks to them.

I informed Benet, politely, but with attempted humor, I would find it difficult to forgive either him or McCabe for breaking the story the way they did. Had the editorial just been published without additional fanfare and sensationalism, the intense media interest would not have developed so explosively, and undoubtedly both Dean Korn and I could have managed it with less disruption to our lives. As it was, I found myself in the front seat of a roller coaster just starting up that first awesome hill, hanging on for dear life.

Overnight the media barrage had gone from local to national. I did an extensive remote television interview for CNN. I talked by phone or met with writers from the *Los Angeles Times, Newsweek, Time* magazine, and *The New York Times*. When *People* magazine called, I requested editorial privilege over what they would write and publish, and when they refused, I decided not to meet with their reporter. *Good Morning America* and *Today* sent satellite trucks to the VA for a live interview at 4:30 in the morning. Slowly I was becoming convinced that the societal issues which had surfaced were very important, not just for me and Stanford's medical school, but for the next generations of women who wanted to be doctors, as well as for those who would become their patients. The president of the Stanford Medical Student Association invited me to an open forum with interested students. I agreed to be there.

My life was completely disrupted. So, I assumed, was Gerry's. I felt I owed him an explanation. After the early morning television appearances I wrote him a short note: "I owe you an apology for the way issues have evolved over the past few days. . . . I did not intend for anything like this to break, especially since you were away. In my dealings with the press I have never named you; your dean is responsible for that disclosure. . . . I know I have not been able adequately to explain to you or to Dean Korn why your day-to-day behavior toward me and many others is so demeaning. I believe you have ingrained behavior patterns to which you are oblivious and which you truly cannot change. I believe that you are not the type of department chair who will be a credit to our department. I am sorry we have these differences of opinion. I wish you the best of luck in your new position and hope the department thrives and prospers."

Stanford's president, Donald Kennedy, called, his first contact since I had resigned more than a week before. He and I have been friends since the early 1960s. His opening question remains imprinted on my brain. "Fran, is this really important?" I quickly thought back to his own personal life. In 1987, he divorced his wife after a marriage of more than thirty years, and a brief time later married a younger woman, a lawyer on his legal staff. It was a very unpopular move with alumni and the university community. When accusations were made that his wedding reception, silk sheets, and antique furniture were improperly paid for with government money, his private life became the object of public ridicule. No wonder he had been quiet. How could he chastise Gerry merely for calling me "honey"? Rather than react with total disbelief and anger at his words, I told him, in a very level tone of voice, that I thought the problem had started with Dean Korn and his misguided selection of Gerry, and, therefore, the dean should be the one to handle the repercussions. Kennedy's instantaneous relief at the unexpected reprieve was relayed over the phone.

The local press continued to look for new angles as follow-up stories appeared. The dean's office was still under siege. Gerry returned from out of town, but remained "unavailable for comment." I was not surprised to learn his silence was at the dean's request. Both men had to believe the first few days of June were but a temporary chaotic aberration disturbing their more predictable, settled worlds—akin to living with diminishing aftershocks following a major earthquake. There was no reason to believe an internecine academic fight would sustain media interest, especially if one side refused to throw any punches. One could just imagine the potential headlines: "The battle of the brain surgeons! Brain docs duke it out!"

Dean Korn, meanwhile, changed tactics with the press, and unwittingly kept the issue alive by doing so. Instinctively he knew Gerry would be a loudmouthed liability were he allowed to meet with the press, but had he unleashed him for a one-on-one confrontation, the dean could have stayed on the periphery of the argument. Instead, he indicated he regretted my resignation, wanted me to consider returning, and would speak to Gerry about my allegations before deciding on the chairmanship. He now admitted the medical school had sexist attitudes, and insensitivity to women and minorities was rampant in the medical profession. Accordingly, the media decided to look inside.

———

Abuse of medical students was the topic of two studies published in 1990.[1] [2] Uninvited and unwanted sexual advances had been experienced by 55–60 percent of the female respondents. Most frequently these were from clinical faculty members or interns and residents. In a 1989 survey by the American Medical Women's Association, 27 percent of practicing women doctors had experienced sexual harassment just within the preceding year.[3] These are alarming numbers, indicating that women are not welcome or even tolerated if they converge on the same playing field where the men have gathered. In fact, a later comprehensive study by the Council on Graduate Medical Education concluded that "gender bias is the single greatest deterrent to women physicians achieving their full potential in every area and aspect of the medical profession and across all stages of medical careers."[4] Women physicians are paid less (both in and outside of academia), are promoted more slowly, and hold very few top leadership positions. The only real cultural change in medicine since 1960 is in the sheer number of women in medical school.

Preclinical educational programs maintain a masculine orientation and the 55-kilogram woman has yet to supplant, substitute, or even gain equal footing with the time-honored male model in the core curriculum. "Women's health" remains fragmented, divided into "reproductive health" and "all other medical problems," without cohesive concern for life cycle changes in health needs or true preventive health for women throughout their lives. In order to really study "women" and their medical afflictions at Stanford, medical students are encouraged to take an elective course—a lecture class called Women and Health Care

1 D. V. Sheehan et al. "A Pilot Study of Medical Student Abuse, *Journal of the American Medical Association*, 1990, 263:533.
2 AAMC Medical School Graduate Questionnaire, Washington, D.C., 1990.
3 S. Lenhart et al. "Gender Bias and Sexual Harassment of AMWA Members in Massachusetts," *Journal of the American Medical Women's Association*, 1991, 46(4):121.
4 Council on Graduate Medical Education, Fifth Report: "Women & Medicine: Women in the Physician Workforce," July 1995.

or a clinical rotation, Women's Health Clerkship. Five students, all female, elected the clerkship in 1996, leaving thirteen vacant slots. The class attracted 61 students, 29 medical students and 32 undergraduates (mostly premeds). Of the 61, eight were men. Only a quarter of this nation's medical schools even offer such electives.

Women physicians continue to be clustered in the lower-paying and lower-prestige areas of medicine. About 60 percent of all women practice in five specialties: family practice, general internal medicine, obstetrics-gynecology, pediatrics, and psychiatry, compared with 40 percent of men. There is real concern that a two-tiered system will result in which women deliver basic but less valued health care, while men continue to populate and prosper in procedure-based specialties in which women are critically underrepresented. Once in place, this top tier may well be increasingly closed to women practitioners in the future.

However, the large infusion of women doctors into primary care ultimately may be very beneficial to patients. In a 1990s study 90 percent of women patients and 25 percent of male respondents felt women's practice styles would improve patient care.[5] Nevertheless, there still are many more men than women practicing medicine, many of whom retain rigid stereotypes they were, and are, taught. A national survey of 2,500 women patients from all socioeconomic backgrounds revealed their increasing dissatisfaction as consumers of health care.[6] A quarter reported they were "talked down" to or "treated like a child," and slightly less than 20 percent felt that a medical complaint was trivialized by being told that it was "all in their head." A disturbing 5 percent reported that a physician had made an offensive sexual remark or inappropriate advance. My male neurosurgical colleagues at Stanford uniformly and without a second thought ad-

5 J. Mandelbaum-Schmidt, "Are Women Physicians Changing the Practice of Medicine?" *MD*, March 1992, 69.
6 Survey of Women's Health. Conducted by Louis Harris and Associates for the Commonwealth Fund, July 1993.

dress their female patients, in all age groups, by their first names; male patients more often, although not always, are "Mr."

By 1991 the nursing profession was changing tiny increment by tiny increment, and had begun to break from the ranks of the impoverished, the belittled, the quietly acquiescent. Technological advances, especially in close monitoring of patients, demanded technical expertise from nurses. A good intensive care nurse, at times, knows far more about a particular patient and his or her needs than does the doctor writing the orders. But, despite this progress, a stereotyped image of the nurse as the doctor's hand-maiden persists, and the professional prestige of a nurse is not even in the same stratosphere as that of a physician.

The scientific research world also has largely ignored women. There are many more male than female research scientists. To date, male scientists have asked the majority of study questions, and the questions have been about men and what ails them. Until 1990 women were routinely omitted from investigational clinical trials, ostensibly because the monthly fluctuation of hormone levels produced too many variables and/or a woman just might be pregnant, putting her fetus at risk. However, many clinical trials are directed at diseases of the aging patient, a time when most women no longer have monthly hormonal changes, and are very thankful they no longer have to worry about pregnancy. Despite the fact that women live years beyond their menopause and that exogenous estrogen and progesterone have been available since the middle of this century, we still have no definitive knowledge as to whether hormone replacement therapy (HRT) is ultimately advantageous or injurious to the aging woman. Clinical investi-gation to resolve these unanswered questions, which, by this time, should be basic medical knowledge, is in its infancy.

Not only is there a void of information about health concerns unique to women, they have also been excluded from studies on health problems known to affect both genders. The human im-munodeficiency virus (HIV) infects both men and women. A con-siderable body of knowledge has been collected since 1980 about

HIV transmission in and between men despite the fact that in most of the world HIV is transmitted by heterosexual contact. However, the first large-scale (and quite recent) study on HIV infection in women was done on *pregnant* women, because the virus is known to cause fetal infection by passing through the placental barrier. The study's concern was for the infected baby, not for the woman.

Aging women suffer from many of the same diseases as men. But women have been invisible, the assumption being that medical regimes that help men are equally applicable to women, despite differences in hormonal makeup, body weight, and surface area. For example, we now know from large-scale clinical trials that an aspirin a day will markedly reduce the number of heart attacks suffered by men. Women were not included as subjects in this study, so the efficacy of aspirin in decreasing the incidence of the number one killer for them remains unknown. It is only within the last five years that the NIH has mandated that researchers include both genders in clinical trials unless there are justifiable compelling reasons to omit one or the other.

Does the medical profession revere men over women because we know more about them? Quite possibly. Would increased knowledge about women, their bodies, and their health, along with a broader research base, give women greater legitimacy in our world? Give our women practitioners a more even footing with male doctors? Only time will tell. But as the media looked inside our peculiar world in the early 1990s it found that woman, as medical student, physician, nurse, patient, scientist, or research subject, clearly was number two in priority and remained vulnerable to abuse by a system which had carefully defined her importance, her role, and, most of all, her limits.

On June 3, Wednesday, in the late afternoon, I met with the students, at their request, at a forum they had organized. The student press estimated attendance at 250 students, fairly evenly divided between men and women and representing well over 50 percent of the entire medical student body. I was astounded by the number; the students were, after all, in the middle of final exams. Also, while I had face and name recognition because I was Senate chair, I was not acquainted with many on an individual basis, so they were not there because of personal friendship. Students served as monitors to prohibit other faculty or members of the administration from attending our gathering.

I gave the students a succinct description of events leading to my resignation, including the impact of the Senate meeting on my thinking. I confessed to having personally participated in perpetuating a sexist climate at their school. For years I had been an "enabler," choosing to ignore sexist insults because no harm was really intended, not realizing that to endure meant to condone. I acknowledged that silence rarely, if ever, has brought about change. It was time to generate some noise.

In response there were expressions of gratitude for my stance, questions about my future, and a comment from a female student who blurted out that Dr. Silverberg had been arrogant, patronizing, and discouraging when she had asked him about spending time on an elective neurosurgical clerkship.

As the hour neared its end, a very articulate male medical student stood up. He turned sideways, leaning on the back of his chair, so he could address the crowd as well as me. "I'm not going to name names, but there's a story that needs to be told about this medical school, some of its faculty, and the administration. I'm not involved but those who are are good friends, and they deserve better than the way they've been treated. Any complaints about sexual harassment are hidden, buried, and ignored by this dean—he either doesn't know how to or doesn't want to handle the problem. Two women medical students have filed two separate formal grievances against a professor in the Department of Medicine having to do with inappropriate sexual come-ons on the part of the professor. They both believe they aren't his first victims, and if Dean Korn has his way and does nothing, they won't be his last. The professor gets away with this stuff time and time again because he's powerful and everyone's too afraid of his influence to stop it. My friends filed their complaints asking that as much as possible they not be identified for obvious reasons having to do with their future careers. They had a couple of meetings early on with the dean and a university lawyer, then nothing. When they inquire where things are, they're fed a bunch of mumbo jumbo about protecting the professor, due process, not wanting the professor to file suit against the university, and all sorts of other garbage. Next week they'll be gone for the summer and the university doesn't need to worry anymore, does it? When they return in the fall, it'll be as if nothing happened; it'll all be forgotten." He turned from the students and faced me directly. "This is what you face in trying to change this culture—it's an arcane society that doesn't want to change and has the power to make sure it doesn't have to. What're you going to do about it?"

I was taken aback by the slap of the gauntlet as it hit the floor, but quickly realized he did not expect a detailed answer from me— all of us were in this together. I knew there were faculty other than Gerry who were guilty of sexist behavior, but had not known of any formal accusations except those filed against Gerry by the three staff members from my own department. Now I realized, in the past, charges of "sexual harassment" against others had also been dismissed. The issue had never been considered important enough for any action by the current, or past, administration.

Suddenly, I understood the intense student interest in my resignation. Because the administration's attention was now dramatically focused on the sexist climate at our school, the students saw an opportunity for these recent events to catalyze change in the status quo.

After the meeting I surreptitiously visited the neurosurgery offices at Stanford. There I found a stack of letters in my mailbox, some from friends, far more from strangers, many envelopes marked "confidential" or "personal." Never having written a fan letter myself, I found it curious that total strangers took the time to write to someone they had never met, and did so without any expectation of receiving an answer in return. These letters continued to pour in for weeks. Phil and I developed the habit of spending the first part of every evening reading the day's correspondence over a glass of wine. Most of the writers, including a surprising number of men, applauded my stand. Often the letters were outpourings of workplace abuse, retribution for blowing the whistle, job termination without cause, and failure of administrative personnel to understand or to act. But some were negative, calling me a man-hater, a rabid feminist, a destructive, vindictive person, a lesbian. A few writers praised Dr. Silverberg's virtues as a person and physician and hoped my ill-conceived actions would not prevent his being awarded the promotion he so richly deserved.

Dean Korn was also receiving mail, some of which was copied to me. To my surprise and delight both Jolie and Luann wrote to him. I had not solicited their letters or even talked to them about resigning.

I also received a letter that had been copied to both Dean Korn and President Kennedy. If the two administrators read it and believed in the basic honesty of the author, they had to be concerned.

Dear Dr. Conley,

This letter is to applaud you in the step you have taken against the medical patriarchy at Stanford Medical Center. This was most likely a difficult decision for you and support is being offered.

I was employed as an RN at Stanford from July 1976 to July 1985. Any nurse who has worked at Stanford has seen or been the direct recipient of chauvinistic behavior. For this reason I am glad you have chosen to take this step and I am appreciative you chose to include behavior directed at nurses by male M.D.s as inappropriate as well.

Although I have not seen names mentioned in the paper,

from experience I can tell you that Dr. Gerald Silverberg was known far and wide to be a touchy-feely pig. Routine, unwanted actions from him included comments, a caress along the backside, even a crotch grab of a nurse bending to get medicines out of a cart. These behaviors were overt, often occurring in the hallway at the hospital as rounds were being made. That these behaviors were seen and taught to be acceptable actions for the medical students, interns, and residents is of no doubt. It is appalling that nurses and female medical students have to put up with these unwanted and unacceptable behaviors.

What is equally appalling is that these behaviors were so overt yet ignorance of their occurrence is being claimed. If Dr. Korn is truly ignorant of these behaviors, he is an oblivious and unfit leader. If Dr. Korn was not ignorant of these behaviors yet chose to do nothing to stop them and, in fact, has chosen to promote them by his choice of a department chair, then he is again an unfit leader and should be removed from his position.

By coming forward and informing the public of the pervasive sexism at Stanford you have also done a great service for the female general public. Those women who may have chosen to go to Stanford for their health care now have the knowledge they need to go to an institution where they will receive care not rooted in sexism.

For all the women for whom you have chosen to take this stand, again I thank you. One should never have to expect that in order to be employed or educated it will be at the cost of human dignity.

Sincerely,

The writer signed her name and provided her address in a northern California city. Phil labeled the letter "a keeper."

———

If life had been as usual, the sheer volume of reading required by the daily quotient of mail would have been difficult to incorporate into twelve-hour workdays. But life was hardly as usual. By the second week in June it became obvious I could not continue to see clinic patients at Stanford—the climate resembled the Antarctic in June. It was not fair to my patients, and it was not fair to the residents caught in the middle of our faculty dispute. My presence at Stanford made the residents quite uncomfortable because it forced them to choose sides. Gerry was not talking to me, and, in our unavoidable brief encounters in the shared work environment, would look straight through me as if I were a transparency. So I informed the staff I would finish those operative cases already scheduled at Stanford through the middle of July, then restrict my practice to the VA until the first of September.

The June 12 edition of the *Campus Report* included letters from two different faculty groups. The first was short and published under the headline: "Many Colleagues Want Conley to Be Asked Back."

> *Editor* Campus Report:
>   *We strongly support Dr. Korn's efforts to reinstate Dr. Frances Conley to the faculty of the Stanford University School of Medicine. We value Dr. Conley as a colleague, and take pride in her presence on the faculty of the Department of Neurosurgery.*

The letter was signed by eleven male and female members of the Biochemistry and Developmental Biology faculties, both basic science disciplines. The headline for the second letter was: "Sexual Harassment: It's Not Just Conley's Issue":

> *Editor,* Campus Report:
>   *The news that Dr. Frances Conley has resigned . . . has shocked and saddened us. Dr. Conley cites a long history of sexism and sexual harassment as the reason for her*

resignation. Many other women on the faculty and staff at Stanford can sympathize, having felt the same pain at various times and to various extents. What particularly disturbs us is the thought that if anyone could withstand such treatment, Dr. Conley could. . . .

This dramatic event should serve to remind us all that harassment of women has not ended. Women still feel distressed by many incidents, each seemingly too trivial to mention but cumulatively devastating. Ambitious women feel their progress restrained by some men's demeaning attitudes and many never reach their legitimate goals. Frances Conley has always been aiming for the top and has reached a very high position. Her action must reflect great pain, which is felt by all of us. If at all possible we urge that she rejoin the faculty. Any ongoing injustice must be thoroughly investigated and righted. The treatment of this case is very important as a sign of the seriousness with which such issues will be dealt with here and elsewhere. This is not just Dr. Conley's problem; it is a problem for all women and men in academic medicine.

The letter was signed by twenty-two women faculty members from throughout the school. I was immensely grateful for the public expression of support. The letters told me I was not alone, and there were many who recognized the pervasiveness of the problem in our academic workplace. I was surprised by how many women immediately labeled my experiences as "sexual harassment." While I had been slow to adopt that thinking, and still found the term lacking in scope, not sufficiently descriptive to encompass its deleterious effect on a woman's career, others had no such qualms. My place of work is so isolated from my peer group, the work itself so narrow, focused, and consuming, I had never before given any thought to whether support was there or would ever be needed. Neurosurgery as a specialty leaves little time for other intellectual pursuits. I had no idea there were women faculty at Stanford in disciplines such as sociology, English, anthropology, business, law, and feminist studies who had researched the gender dynamics I was caught up in and could have been of incredible help had I known enough to reach out to them.

When the two campus letters were published, my life was so frantic from the media onslaught I failed to capitalize on a marvelous source of power this number of faculty represented. In retrospect I should have invited faculty, especially women faculty, to meet for a frank discussion about the climate at their medical school and university, and gathered ideas for making our place of employment more receptive and happier for all. United we might have galvanized a sense of urgency behind evolutionary change. Divided and unorganized, we were no threat to those with power to maintain the status quo.

For the entire month of June media coverage of "the Stanford story of sexism" continued virtually unabated. *Nightline* sent a producer to me, I did a long interview for NPR and a segment for *20/20*. Gerry was still "unavailable for comment," so only one side, mine, received attention, and almost uniformly it was remarkably positive. If the press was searching my life for deviant behavior, they were disappointed. My life consisted of work, a little running and javelin throwing, minimal creativity, and no scandal.

Interest in issues of "sexual harassment" in the workplace broadened to include all working women and their varied workplaces. The *San Jose Mercury News* established a "hot line" and invited women to call and share stories with them. A few weeks later they published an anthology of women's employment experiences culled from 126 letters and phone calls they had received. Stories from police officers, telephone linespeople, secretaries, teachers, firefighters, veterinarians resonated with my story and included the injurious effect of sexism on an individual's ability to perform as optimally as possible.

I did not know how to handle the quasi-"celebrity" status that enveloped me, and I felt quite ambivalent about it. From the intense local publicity, both on television and in the print media, strangers recognized me, some even asked for autographs, others just to shake my hand. Mostly, I found the attention embarrassing, albeit tinged with a sense of adventure along with some vulnerability.

While many professionals seek media recognition to enhance their value, for an academic, courting the media is not considered proper. I had broken the unwritten rules by writing the opinion piece, and continued to do so by granting interviews. Of course, the rules make no sense. In general, academics love the attention media gives them and are envious of those who succeed in garnering a positive slant to their endeavors. At the same time, snide comments from colleagues are embarrassing and one dare not let the limelight silhouette one's shadow for any but a few precious moments. A little is permissible, but constant coverage is considered feckless and the worst possible form of self-aggrandizement. Ordinarily, academic institutions control media access quite rigidly. Spin doctors in university news bureaus or public relations offices are paid to accentuate the positive and make the negative positive as well. Damage control is also their responsibility.

However, circumstances in mid-1991 were not favorable for Stanford's media group. Its publicity gurus had been assaulted without respite for most of the prior twelve months trying to explain and excuse the $200 million debt the university allegedly owed the government for years of overcharges and false charges made to research budgets. Their task became more difficult after an abysmal performance in the winter by President Donald Kennedy and his legal staff in Washington, D.C., before Representative John Dingell's investigative congressional subcommittee—

and national television cameras. Repair work on the university's image and reputation was crucial and represented a major focus for the press corps at the time I resigned. Plans for a huge centennial celebration to take place at the end of September 1991 had been finalized, and alumni donors were expected generously to forgive and forget not only the charges against but also the arrogance shown by their alma mater.

University media folk underestimated the amount of sustained interest there would be about societal issues of workplace sexism and sexual harassment. My story was especially compelling because of its setting within the revered medical profession, because it had happened at one of the nation's most prestigious medical schools, and because it involved "brain surgeons." The typical university squelch machine failed to materialize—no effort was made to control media access to me, or mine to them. I had sinned royally by going to the press, but knew the media had helped to open a hidden part of the medical school culture, one that affected lives beyond the professionals who worked there (in particular, patients). Because the story made national news so rapidly and sensationally, by continuing to work with the press I was provided with an opportunity to openly confront traditional assumptions about our environment and might, I thought, accelerate change in attitudes and behavior. The press remained unfettered for an unusual length of time, effectively preventing David Korn from completing his desired agenda in a timely manner.

7 On Wednesday morning, June 26, the *San Francisco Chronicle* carried a front-page story headlined: "Stanford Files Sex Charge Against Professor. Harassment Accusations by 2 Students in Medical School." All of the other peninsula papers also ran their version, and I finally learned the identity of the professor the students had challenged.

The news revitalized the media's interest, and I fielded a number of phone calls that morning asking for my thoughts, but my only knowledge came from the media itself. Two female medical students had filed formal grievances against Dr. Mark Perlroth, professor of clinical medicine in cardiology, over two separate incidents of allegedly harassing behavior. In the first case, because of his own personal attraction to a student, he refused to consider her application for a teaching assistantship and continued to pursue her through repeated telephone, written, and personal contact, despite her requests that he leave her alone. In the second case, Dr. Perlroth, who is married and has children, was accused of lowering the score on the exam of a female student, thus forcing her to communicate with him about retaking the exam or the entire course. The student met with him alone in his office and claimed he inappropriately had channeled the conversation into personal subjects, asking her a series of increasingly intimate questions, including queries with sexual overtones.

Mark Perlroth and I had joined the faculty at about the same time, but we had very infrequent contact. A former medical student, who undoubtedly had interacted with him much more than I ever did, wrote to President Kennedy on June 26: "In 1976, when I was a first-year medical student, I called Dr. Perlroth's behavior to the attention of the very highest levels of the medical school. I expressed my concerns again in 1977, and since then had heard nothing. I, therefore, assumed that the authorities of the medical school had taken care of the problem. I am now affronted and disgusted to find out that his behavior has continued damaging untold numbers of female medical students over the past 15 years. If no one had tried to blow the whistle it would be more understandable, but I think that the scrutiny since 1976 should have surely been better than it was. I am expecting to see very strong action taken to sanction Dr. Perlroth."

The former student who wrote the letter is a friend of mine and is now a general surgeon practicing in Palo Alto. The copy she sent me opened my eyes to the real scope and depth of the societal illness the students and I had broken into. How and why do academic medical centers provide a base of operation for people like Perlroth? The fact is that in universities there is a covenant of secrecy and silence. Because one brother will not chastise another, a harasser is provided with privacy as well as unfettered opportunity. And failure to apply meaningful public sanctions in response to behavioral deviancy sets the stage for repetition of the behavior—often multiple times.

The formal charge against Dr. Perlroth was issued from the president's office. The alleged episodes were labeled "professional misconduct" in standard university language, and President Kennedy proposed that Dr. Perlroth be suspended from duty without pay for a period of one year. The term "professional misconduct" covers a variety of transgressions—plagiarism, violations of health and safety, improper use of funds from granting agencies, illegal consulting practices, sexual harassment. Professor Mark Perlroth had heard the two words before, but the university had never allowed them to tarnish his ascending career. He had a legal right to contest the grievances and request a hearing before the University Advisory Board, something he and his attorney promptly did.

According to news reports, Dr. Perlroth vigorously denied the charges against him, and he further criticized the university for making them public before the outcome of his hearing. He placed the blame for the university's actions squarely on my shoulders. He felt he was a "scapegoat for the damaging publicity surrounding the resignation of a popular neurosurgeon a month ago amid claims of sexism at the school"(*Peninsula Times Tribune*, June 26, 1991), and, according to him, "Kennedy went public with the complaints against him in reaction to the notoriety given to Conley's resignation and to the climate of scandal that has dogged Stanford in the wake of investigations of overcharges for federal research" (*San Francisco Chronicle*, June 26, 1991). Dr. Perlroth's comments suggested that he believed that without my resignation and the ensuing publicity over sexism and sexual harassment, the charges against him certainly would not have been made public and might even have been dismissed. Most likely he was speaking from past experience, and, as such, was delivering a message the medical students had feared—that grievances of this type could be trivialized, buried, and forgotten.

In part of a prepared statement, Dr. Perlroth declared, "I chose to assert my right to defend myself. The accusations are creating a hostile environment by words and not deeds. There is no exchange of favors for a position"(*San Francisco Chronicle*, June 26, 1991). Dr. Perlroth's defense rested on his First Amendment rights to freedom of speech, a defense Dean Korn would support. This despite direct conflict with wording in the Sexual Harassment Policy in place at Stanford University since 1981:

"[harassment] might be described generally as repeated and un-wanted sexual behavior, such as . . . verbal comments or sugges-tions."

I remember thinking that morning, "Hooray for the univer-sity, and especially President Kennedy—maybe he's finally real-ized this issue is important." Being a professor does not entitle one to gratuitous sexual gratification or even being a sexist boor. Sidelined by all the participants, however, is the real question of whether or not the two female complainants, working hard to become doctors, had been taken seriously as students by a teacher who had a rather solemn obligation to do so. Also, I am not sure anyone considered, or even cared, whether their tawdry experi-ence at Stanford would have a negative impact on their subse-quent careers as medical professionals.

But without the two cases against Perlroth, the students might have registered only marginal interest in my resignation. The issue of sexual harassment became a hot item for our community and the media because the school had two complaints to handle si-multaneously. With student involvement a large vocal army col-lected and strength in numbers gave considerable credibility to the message that it was time for a culture change at our medical school.

Any institution of higher education has, in place, legal mecha-nisms for dispute management as well as resolution. Stanford is no different. The minute legal action is instigated or even threat-ened, the university assumes a well-rehearsed posture, employing a style of cover-up with which it has considerable experience as well as expertise. Dr. Perlroth had expected the traditional insti-tutional silence to be maintained while legal machinations ran their lengthy course, knowing that passage of time would dull both memory and interest. The publicity that had erupted was unexpected and unwelcome.

By contrast, in Gerry's situation, the legal office was reduced to an effete nonentity because it had no formal complaint demanding its attention. Many times various people asked me when I would file or if I had already filed a grievance or a lawsuit. My plan did not include legal action or filing a formal grievance, as neither addressed my concern. I resigned over a poor choice, a sexist choice, on the part of the dean for executive leadership, a complaint not covered by law or university statute. If I had an actionable case against Gerry for sexism or sexual harassment, I had equally actionable cases against a number of others. Gerry and the university were caught in a spotlight of intense and continuing media scrutiny about the pervasive sexism poisoning a world-renowned medical school, a fact crystallized in the minds of many by the addition of the Perlroth case. My filing a lawsuit or grievance would have rapidly silenced the press and given Stanford a far more manageable situation.

I also knew from personal experience, having been both a plaintiff and a defendant in two different lawsuits, that an adversarial legal system induces polarization and quashes the possibility for friendly resolution. The two sides are drawn, contact between warring factions is prohibited, dialogue is artificially constrained by rules governing evidence, and attorneys run one's life. In this situation, I did not want to inhibit an exchange of ideas. I hoped medical center personnel would talk about their workplaces, discuss sexism, sexual harassment, and job and educational discrimination. For far too long the medical world has denied outright that there is any inequity between men and women. If women understand the issues and men do not, they should talk to each other about what constitutes equality and what is acceptable conduct and what is not, and why. Silence has always been one of women's worst enemies. I thought this was an opportune time for women to be open and articulate about what their professional worlds were really like.

There had been no communication between the dean and me since my letter to him written in the midst of the initial media blitz. However, a week prior to the press release about the Perlroth grievances, I had received a confidential memo from him stating, in part, "I do not for a moment doubt the sincerity of your protest or the seriousness of the issues you are addressing." Then he explained his position. According to Dean Korn, gender insensitivity, sexism, and sexual harassment were "distinct and different both in their nature and in the kinds of responses that can be developed appropriately to respond to them. The responses must be different for the different categories of offense." He wrote further, "Gender insensitivity issues are not much different in kind from the insensitivities that have been debated here and on campuses across the country in the last year, largely driven from concerns with ethnic and multicultural diversity. In those debates . . . issues of freedom of expression have clashed head on with issues of personal debasement and effrontery. . . . I am very concerned about efforts to truncate freedom of expression on a university campus by statute or regulation." He ended by writing, "I also agree with you that our profession, as well as our institution, continues to exhibit offensive stereotypic patterns of ideation and behavior that reflect generations of white male dominance and become increasingly inappropriate with every passing year. Finally, let me indicate that although you have given me many reasons to believe that your decision to resign your faculty position is final, I would be happy to talk with you about your decision and your future plans at your request."

There was still hope. In response to pressure from the media, faculty, students, and the general public, the dean had extended an invitation to discuss my future, if any, at Stanford University School of Medicine. However, I had no intention of altering my plans to leave in September unless a national search for the chair of my department was reopened.

The content of the memo gave me insight into the dean's thinking and clearly outlined the conundrum the academy has wrestled with for years: Is verbal harassment or hate speech protected by the First Amendment? Is behavior best controlled by legal sanctions or by social pressure, or a combination of both? Does the definition of "sexual harassment" include a hostile environment—one created by persistent verbal diminishment based on gender or race? There is a potential clash between prohibition of harassment and the protection of free speech. There is also a potential clash between harassing speech and pursuit of happiness if an education and a career define happiness for those who are forced out of an environment made "hostile" by spoken comments. Protected speech makes oppression possible and causes pain. It is just as apparent, however, that restrictive speech codes will not alter an ingrained mind-set about the basic inferiority of women or convert the medical profession, or law, or business, or educational institutions into benign places where all have equal opportunity. On that, Dean Korn and I were in agreement. After reading his memo, I had called his office for an appointment to meet with him.

Prior to the meeting I sought advice from a good friend of many years, Professor David Kuechle at Harvard. He teaches negotiation and crisis management, and also is an attorney. He told me this meeting basically would provide information and not much more. I should avoid confrontation and let the dean do the majority of the talking. Kuechle suggested I try to determine, if possible, where Korn was being pressured and by whom. What was the dean's strategic plan for his, my, and Gerry's future?

The meeting was on June 27. I was on time, and Dean Korn did not keep me waiting. His office, large enough for pacing, was orderly and tastefully decorated in an understated fashion. Slightly to the left as one entered was a small circular table with four straight-backed chairs, an arrangement designed for intimacy and to reduce the hierarchical distance between players. That is where we sat. But maintaining eye contact, at least with me, was difficult for him.

Our guarded discussion covered the financial health (or illness) of the school, the intrusive qualities of the media, and our divergent views about Gerry's suitability for appointment to an executive leadership position. The dean had received many letters from other neurosurgeons, faculty, and patients praising Gerry for being a wonderful surgeon, physician, and person (Korn did not mention any negative letters), and he did not regard his choice as inappropriate at all. I was truly dismayed by his lack of vision. Was the dean trying to convince me my intimate observations of Gerry's unattractive conduct spanning some twenty-five years were in error, or worse, should be forgotten, even forgiven? I acknowledged I could not expect him to fully understand Gerry's behavior and how embarrassing it was. My only request was that he reopen the national search. Let Gerry remain in the running, if he wished, but judge him against other candidates, especially in terms of leadership skills. If he emerged as the best person after a legitimate search, I would still leave but at that point I would have no grounds for complaint.

The dean responded curtly that the search had been stopped. Then he looked directly at me for the first time and asked what I thought Gerry would do if he was not given the job. It suddenly occurred to me the dean might have grave personal concerns about Gerry. Did Gerry have grounds for a breach of contract lawsuit? In California, verbal contracts can be binding. Just what had been promised, and when? If a legitimate search was conducted, I knew Gerry, who was somewhat underqualified by academic standards, would suffer by comparison with many of the other neurosurgeons interested in the job. He might not make the final slate of names offered by the search committee. Thus, if David had promised the job to him, one way he could definitely keep that promise was by stopping the search. Financial pressures had become a convenient excuse to do just that.

I did not answer his question directly, telling Korn I had no idea what Gerry would do, but that my department deserved to know who was out there and that Stanford should uphold its long tradition of promoting "only the very best."

Korn was not listening. Instead he told me that over the next week or so he intended to conduct an inquiry into some of the issues I had raised about Gerry. If his inquiries failed to uncover any disturbing features, he planned to finalize Gerry's appointment as chair with the Executive Committee at their July meeting.

I asked, "What if you do find disturbing behavior?"

After a long pause, he said he might consider reopening a limited search (whatever that would be) and appointing another interim acting chair. September 1 was not very far away, so I asked what he wanted me to do with my laboratories. Because research space was so valuable, I knew they would be completely dismantled as soon as I left, and the space allocated to others.

The immediacy of his response startled me: "Please do your best to keep them intact." I knew my laboratories would be very important were he to reopen the search. The research space and equipment I had acquired and still controlled represented a research empire. Even if I were still on the faculty, my facility would constitute a prime resource for a new chair to develop a more extensive research program for the Neurosurgery Department. Thus my laboratories would be an important part of the dean's package in any future negotiations with chair candidates.

I told him I would try. We shook hands cordially but realized very little had been accomplished.

Both my lawyer, John Tyndall, and Dave Kuechle had advised me to keep a "paper trail" documenting all contact with both Gerry and members of the administration, just in case legal action might be necessary in the future. So I typed a list of the points the dean and I had covered in our discussion and sent it to him with the request he "let me know where our recollections are divergent and/or things I have neglected to include."

He rapidly dictated a confidential memo in return, stating the list was accurate with regard to substance, but contained some innuendos he felt the need to challenge. He has always been more comfortable and better at expressing himself in writing. "We differ in respect to the gravity of specific offenses and the burden of proof required to justify official reprimand or punishment. . . . We might both agree that certain kinds of behavior are indeed unacceptable, but it is my view that a punitive response to such unacceptable behavior must be based on a robust body of evidence. Allegations that cannot be substantiated simply won't do. I am proceeding with my inquiry . . . and I would like to resolve this matter upon my return in the latter part of July. Once the resolution has been decided, I believe it will be up to you to determine what next steps you might wish to initiate."

The dean left a couple of days later on a trip to Asia, with plans to return the third week in July. After rereading his memo I remember thinking, "He still just doesn't get it." Of course the dean had an absolute right to require a "robust body of evidence," knowing that any punitive action taken by someone in his visible position would be subject to intense scrutiny. If the dean had promised the chair position to Gerry, to withdraw it now would represent punishment for behavior Gerry, and quite possibly the dean, had rarely, if ever, questioned. I thought it would be much less punitive to reopen the search, visibly keeping Gerry as a viable, and visible, candidate. Then Korn would not be seen as abandoning Gerry, but at the same time would signal an appropriate concern over the broader issues I had raised. David Korn had given himself three weeks for an "inquiry" to be conducted—plenty of time, I thought, for him to collect a "robust body of evidence," if he looked in the right places.

My resignation and the media had put Gerry's appointment on a temporary hold. Initially Gerry did not appear at all worried. It was as if David Korn were constantly reassuring him that with time all would quiet down, life would return to normal, and he would get his chairmanship. To everyone around him Gerry vigorously denied ever having asked me to go to bed with him. He thought he remembered another resident who used to do that to me. Joe Andrus, the junior faculty member who spent part of his time at the VA, reported that Gerry was quite jovial, laughing loudly and accepting the plaudits of male friends, who, confused, would hail him with "You old devil, you—I wish someone would harass me!" When asked to submit the title of his presentation for a scientific society meeting to be held in September, Gerry told the planners he would talk about "Sexual Harassment at Stanford," and the printed program I received for the meeting officially carried that title.

Prior to leaving town, David Korn announced his intent to establish and fund an office for Women in Medicine and the Medical Sciences, and also hired a professional consulting firm, schooled in cultural diversity matters, to conduct a series of workshops, group meetings, and retreats for various faculty constituencies. It would all begin in the fall quarter. The dean's idea was to import "sensitivity" and imprint tolerance on the majority for minorities. He felt the faculty could benefit from direction in those skills and techniques necessary to modify "the culture of an institution to assure that persons of different cultural traditions feel welcome." The *Campus Report* covered the intent and activities of the dean's office in considerable detail, and gave the dean kudos for his exceptional insight and forceful response. I laughed, and wondered how, with the financial woes that daily consumed him, Korn planned to pay for all these energetic programs of good intent. But no matter how much money was spent, the programs were doomed to failure unless there was unequivocal, genuine, hands-on support from him.

A few days after my conversation with the dean I received a disquieting phone call at the VA from Jolie. Shortly after I resigned, Jolie was asked to meet with the Human Resources Office about her experiences in my department, which she did. Afterward, she had been contacted by a man purporting to be from "Stanford University Human Resources" who asked her to meet with him and provide a taped statement. She did not recognize the name, told him she would get back to him, and shrewdly called Human Resources. They also did not recognize the name;

the man was not a Stanford employee. Jolie asked Human Resources to return his phone call for her and find out who he was.

It turned out the man was a private investigator hired by Gerry and his attorney. The investigator's assignment was to talk to people who might have damaging things to say about Gerry. When confronted by Human Resources about the detective's misleading characterization as a Stanford employee, Gerry told them he had not authorized the private investigator to misrepresent himself. Jolie had called to ask if the private detective had contacted me and, if not, to warn me. Jolie also told me phones at the Stanford neurosurgery offices, where she first tried to reach me, were being answered with "Dr. Conley no longer works here and we don't know where she is or how to reach her." I was rapidly becoming a nonbeing. Inexorably, the conflict was escalating.

Within a week after talking with Jolie, I arrived at my VA office one morning to find it in a state of disarray far in excess of my usual messiness. It appeared whoever had been rummaging around had been interrupted and departed abruptly. Anyone could have obtained admittance to the office. Security personnel were not acquainted with the entire staff and did not always ask for identification before unlocking doors. On any given day, many people visited the surgical suite, some of whom were transient professionals rotating back and forth between the VA and the medical center. I remember not being at all surprised by the incident and resigned myself to rearranging my office, knowing if anything was missing, my attorney, John Tyndall, possessed copies of everything that could be construed as sensitive. Breaking into an office at a VA hospital is a federal offense, but nothing of material value appeared to be missing and I did not report it, not wishing to give our departmental conflict increased visibility. On a personal level it was most disturbing to know some stranger had been in my office. His (or her) presence was a violation of my space and, thus, of me. I was equally disturbed by the thought of espionage occurring in the reputedly revered, benign, compassionate, caring world of academic medicine.

It had been only five weeks since I resigned—it seemed more like five months or even years. On July 4, Phil and I left for a four-day mini vacation to throw in a Master's javelin competition. It felt so good to get away. Over the preceding month I had lost ten pounds. I was absolutely exhausted, and I slept as well as I ever have away from home. The interlude was all too brief.

On returning, I was unceremoniously jerked back to the reality of patients, surgery, a new resident, interviews, phone calls, many, many letters, a deposition, Medical Faculty Senate committee meetings, and the Advisory Board. Nothing seemed right. Rita, my secretary at the VA, asked me to pick up a ream of letterhead Stanford stationery, which I used for any non-VA correspondence. All faculty were included on the letterhead with both Stanford and VA affiliations listed. I found I had been expunged from the letterhead completely, from both institutions, even though my resignation was not effective for another month and a half. I marveled how rapidly sixteen years of a professional career could disappear.

Despite my department doing its best to deny my presence, people at the medical school were talking—about sexism, harassment, inequality of opportunity. The talk forced thinking, and thinking brought memories and with it guilt—for some. Over the years, others had shared clandestine stories with me about many high-ranking, prestigious doctors on our faculty—Christmas parties, where too much alcohol led to a secretary or female house officer finding herself alone with a faculty member in his office, followed by forced attentions and ripped clothing. Furtive looks were shared, as the unanswered question was asked, "Who's going to share secrets about me, with whom, and when?" Human nature would suggest those capable of expressing concern and camaraderie with me during those difficult days in June and July had nothing to hide. Those who shunned me were wondering when the skeletons in their own closets would start to dance. Phil and I informally started "counting noses"—which acquaintances believed in "the cause" and which did not.

I was asked to speak at a breakfast meeting of a local Rotary Club and a dinner meeting of a Stanford women's alumni group held at a local restaurant. I told them about Stanford Medical School and described my world within that world, the Senate meeting, the forum with the students. After my presentation at the dinner meeting, a woman from the back of the crowded room shouted, "How can we help you?" I was at a total loss as to how I should answer her. Subliminally, I was aware, from observing the political scene, that in the United States the woman who does not fit the romantic stereotype of a female has difficulty mustering public support, so I had never sought it. However, here was a room filled to capacity with supportive women, and I never thought about using them, or any ad hoc constituency, such as the faculty women, for "help." I had been away from women, collectively, for so long, I had not considered the force and source of power their numbers might have represented.

I also felt considerable ambivalence about escalating the conflict by involving others. I had always operated independently and, to date, had done just fine. Also, my generation of women generally had not learned to work with each other, but rather to compete with each other, especially for attention, especially from men. I was not socialized to ask for help from women, had not learned to trust them, and had no idea what type of help I could expect.

While the dean was away I received a few interesting and unexpected phone calls. The CEO of Stanford Hospital, Ken Bloem, called to ask if I was interested in being considered for Chief of Staff of the hospital. I was very intrigued; the position represented an unanticipated reprieve from impending unemployment. It was also comforting to realize I had not been totally ostracized. The Chief of Staff is a highly visible person in our medical world and one who reports to the hospital CEO. As Chief of Staff I would maintain a faculty appointment and ties to my medical education, but have the chance to decide whether I enjoyed administrative work. As an added plus, a real opportunity to use some of my business education would be part of the job. Under the right conditions it would be the perfect position for me. But was I being bought off?

As the top hospital administrator, Ken Bloem had quickly earned the respect of the medical community as a smart, shrewd operator, one who had innovative ideas and a clear vision about the future direction of medicine. I knew he and David Korn were not working well together, but also that Korn would have to ratify Ken's choice for Chief of Staff. Appointment of me as Chief of Staff would not help Korn in any way, except to maintain one of his few tenured female faculty. Korn would never agree to such a visible appointment for me unless he could use it to his advantage, and there was one possible scenario that was totally unacceptable. He might demand a trade-off: Chief of Staff position for me, neurosurgery chair for Gerry. If I became Chief of Staff and withdrew opposition to Gerry's appointment, those who had accused me of using the charge of sexism to advance my own position would believe they had been correct. I told Ken I was interested but that the two appointments had to be treated as mutually exclusive events and could not be coupled in any way.

I was also contacted by the Equal Employment Opportunity Commission (EEOC). Sally Hawthorne, the district director of the San Francisco office, called to request a meeting. I told her I was not inclined to file any complaint with the EEOC. "No matter," she told me. "The publicity has given us ample ammunition whether or not you ever sign a complaint." Apparently the commission could institute enforcement action on its own if a significant number of gender, race and/or age-based cases had been filed against a single institution. When sufficient evidence surfaced to substantiate possible illegal discrimination, the commission could file charges, without an individual complainant, assuming burden of proof and all costs of the investigation. The EEOC had the power of subpoena, but was not likely to file charges unless there was plenty of evidence. Sally Hawthorne's request was actually a command. Her office had received numerous complaints from Stanford employees, mostly women, about their work environments, and she was considering filing a class action suit against the university for its employment practices. Our calendars did not match until the end of July.

8 While the dean was still away Morgan Idlewild, a recent Ph.D. graduate in neurobiology, and a friend of mine, phoned to say that Gerry had just offered my VA laboratories to him. I was shocked.

Morgan's wife, Professor Corinne Spitz, Ph.D., is one of the premier neurobiologists in the world. She had told me earlier she might be leaving Stanford. I had heard rumors she was unhappy because Stanford would not give an academic appointment in neurobiology to Morgan. Other institutions were eager to hire both of them, and Corinne had informed Dean Korn before he left on his trip of their intention to move north across the bay to Stanford's archrival, the University of California at Berkeley. Dean Korn had asked her to delay her final decision until he returned.

I shared my fears with Morgan that he and Corinne were being used as pawns by Gerry to gain favor with the dean in order to guarantee closure on his chairmanship. If Gerry saved Corinne by offering employment and laboratory space to Morgan, the dean would be eternally grateful. But Gerry was offering a gift of something he did not own or even control. Unlike at Stanford, research space at the VA is not assigned by clinical service or department, but on the basis of an individual's research funding. Not knowing the research game, Gerry was unaware neurosurgery did not own my research space and thus it was not his to give away. The dean probably could have finessed the federal system and made VA Research Administration give the space to Morgan, but Gerry could not. Gerry might also have suddenly recognized the value of the laboratories to the dean, were he to reopen the search. By giving them away, he could remove one big item from a contract package, and push Korn firmly in the direction of confirming his appointment.

Evidently, in the spring, Gerry had made an earlier offer of employment to Morgan but had never mentioned my laboratories as part of the deal. He and Corinne rejected Gerry's offer because there was no identified, committed research space for him. They also had concerns about continued support from Gerry because his was an acting position and a new permanent chair would have the right to terminate Morgan immediately. In negotiations with Corinne at that time, the dean had tried to reassure her everything would be fine for both of them. They really did not know whether they could believe him because he had just opened the national search for the neurosurgery chair position.

I told Morgan with a bit of anger, and some sadness over a lost opportunity, that my laboratories did not belong to Gerry. Had I known earlier that he needed research space I would have bent over backward to accommodate him—Gerry had never told me he was planning to develop a position for Morgan within our department. Now Morgan and Corinne had to make a decision about their collective future by the end of July, and the availability of my laboratories was integral to that decision.

In anticipation of his return, I scribbled a handwritten note to Dean Korn, just to remind him about unfinished business: "Per your letter of July 3, I look forward to learning the results of your inquiry, and would hope the results of same would be available sometime this week or in the early part of next. Thanks."

I was more than a little uneasy. Because Dean Korn had been away, he himself could not have conducted any "inquiry," and I had not been contacted by anyone else asking whether I had information about Gerry, sexual harassment, or sexism. I was almost certain there had been no inquiry, and wondered if Korn had ever intended to conduct one. The school was in the middle of academic summer doldrums. Day after perfect day the sky was blue, the air warm, the breezes mild, welcome and capricious—weather for barbecues, the ocean, hiking, biking, running, and swimming, not for dealing with contentious issues. I was afraid Dean Korn, believing the Conley mess would disappear during his three-week absence, still hoped to push Gerry's appointment through without any inquiry, and would do so at a time when students were not around and his executives were settled into the soothing complacency of daily California sunshine.

A regularly scheduled meeting of the Executive Committee was on my calendar for Friday, July 26. The agenda for the meeting was totally benign. As Senate chair I was expected to attend, and I did, deliberately, in order to retain visibility and to remind the executive group I was still around with unfinished business—business that was not the sole prerogative of the dean. David Korn greeted me with a neutral nod, and soon passed me a brief note suggesting that he and I meet later. It would be best, the note said, if I did not attend the Executive Session (when promotions and appointments are considered and all ancillary personnel are asked to leave). Gerry was out of town, which the dean apparently knew. I assumed the major agenda item for the session would be Gerry's appointment, and I left the meeting in good humor amid an atmosphere of friendship on the part of those executives in attendance.

I heard nothing of what had been resolved at the Executive Session on that Friday. By Monday I was extremely anxious to learn what had happened. So I called one of the department chairs, a good friend of mine. He positively chortled. The dean had admitted Gerry was a bit of a "scuzz-ball," but still felt the appointment was in the best interest of my department and the school. My understanding is that stories were shared, some probably coming from Lois Sweet, chair of the Department of Developmental Biology, who had been fielding phone calls from women ever since my resignation. My friend told me the dean had received a real dressing-down and was admonished by his executives that he had blundered badly in his decision to appoint Gerry to head my department. They were especially critical of the dean for failing to ask their advice in advance of his deciding on the chair position. The group must have been heavily influenced by the presence of the two female department chairs. Also, I was well known to this crowd, as I had been an integral player for the past two years—they knew I was usually rational. In an open forum with considerable social pressure for conformity, none of the male executives were willing to go on record in front of the others as condoning sexist, insensitive actions toward women, which was how Gerry's behavior had been characterized. At the end of their discussion, the executives had unanimously recommended to Dean Korn that he reopen the national search and do whatever was necessary for me to rejoin the faculty.

As the phone conversation progressed, my emotions reached an all-time high. I was elated, ecstatic, euphoric, energized. My crazy negative world had finally flip-flopped to positive. Suddenly all the agony and unhappiness of the past two months had been worthwhile. I was going to win after all. His executives had endorsed me, not Gerry, and told the dean I was worth keeping.

The large headline on the front page of the *San Francisco Chronicle* on July 30 read: "Stanford's President to Resign." In smaller headline print: "Kennedy, plagued by billing scandal, tells trustees he will step down next year." It was no longer important that the president had chosen to absent himself from the turmoil at the medical school. The same morning Sally Hawthorne from the EEOC called to say she could not make our scheduled meeting; could we try again the first week in August? The delay presented no problem. Given what appeared to be a reversal of circumstances in my favor, I certainly did not wish to unnecessarily antagonize a dean who might finally do what should have been done in the first place. I could tell the EEOC that attitudes had changed and the future of our school looked bright indeed, especially for its women and minority members. Stanford would earn itself a prominent spot in history for changing the face of the medical profession.

Over the next few days, I was a little surprised by continued silence from the dean's office. But at least I now knew he did not always respond to events rapidly. Then, late Friday afternoon, a week after his executives had failed him, the dean's secretary called to say that Dean Korn wished to talk with me. I anticipated having a full, complicated agenda to discuss and suggested the dean and I set a face-to-face meeting for early the next week, rather than talking on the phone. I could hear her relaying my request. Suddenly the dean grabbed the phone. He was very angry. In a loud, strident voice he told me he had reopened the national search, for whatever that would be worth. Also, he was incredibly unhappy with the course of events, and that it had been the *executives* who felt reopening the search was necessary. With increasing frenzy and rapidity of speech, the pitch of his voice rising higher and higher, he added that he hoped I realized all hell was breaking loose and that it was entirely my fault.

I could not help but answer his anger with my own: "David, don't yell at me! You brought this on yourself—you've only yourself to blame! Look, I don't think this is a good time for us to talk. Can we meet sometime next week?" We set the meeting for 10:30 a.m., Tuesday, August 6.

I later learned Gerry had just left the dean's office and, not unexpectedly, was furious. Dr. Silverberg spent that afternoon and the entire weekend commandeering anyone he could, including all the residents, to write letters to the dean on his behalf.

I called Dave Kuechle at Harvard and told him about my brief conversation with the dean. His first question was, "Why do you suppose he's so angry?"

"Dave, I don't know. You tell me. I can make some guesses . . ."

"Go ahead."

"I think Korn probably has promised the chair position to Gerry, and until now has been reassuring him he would keep his promise. Now suddenly, he's had to recant—his executives have forced the issue. Why hasn't the dean contacted me until now? I think he's had to figure out how to handle Gerry, and probably didn't do it very well."

Kuechle wanted to know what the dean had to lose.

"Gerry isn't exactly a nice person when he doesn't get his way. My bet is he's threatened the dean with a breach of contract lawsuit. Either that or he's got some dirt on the dean, which wouldn't surprise me either. Gerry may well know something from his past and I don't believe he's above blackmail, especially when his entire career's on the line. If he goes down, he'll take his buddy with him. Christ, he may sue me too."

Dave Kuechle, ever cautious, had some reservations about my thinking. The dean's liability was now shared with his executives, so his vulnerability in any legal action was markedly reduced. A lawsuit against the school would be very difficult for Gerry to win, and legal action against me would risk exposing himself to embarrassing questions.

He suggested I support the dean and congratulate him for having made a courageous decision. I should offer to help achieve our common goal of a culture change directed at reducing sexism and racism at the medical school. Although the magnitude of his anger frightened me, I must refrain from answering anger with more anger. If I could avoid threats, such as using the EEOC, the ultimate result would be more positive.

I went to the meeting Tuesday morning feeling very optimistic and clear about the role I should play. The search had been re-opened and the only uncertainty I faced was whether I wanted to, or could, rejoin the faculty if the dean were to make such an offer. If the Chief of Staff position was extended, it would be delightful to be back on the faculty. I would be an inactive member of the Neurosurgery Department, reporting to Ken Bloem, and my faculty appointment would be completely out of the dean's hands. Also, I would not have to deal with the negativity, hostility, and acrimony that would exist in my department were I to come back to my former position with Gerry still around.

I was in the process of awkwardly congratulating the dean on his "courageous decision" when he interrupted me to say that things had changed. Circumstances were no longer as they had been on Friday. David Korn was clearly uncomfortable, but at the same time in control. Obviously he had been thinking and planning since his angry phone call Friday afternoon. Although we were seated at the circular table, the conversation was one-sided and, as usual, without eye contact. He told the ceiling that while he had reopened the search, it would not be an active one. His words suddenly made me very uneasy. I stared at him, my body immobile, frozen.

Then Korn launched into the main thrust of what he had to say, speaking as if he had rehearsed the soliloquy a number of times. His executives had acted in haste, and had been terribly naive in their failure to understand the public repercussions of the advice they had given him. Many of them had phoned during the week to say they wished to change their stance, that Gerry had been judged unfairly, and certainly been denied any sem-blance of due process. While some worrisome material had sur-faced during the discussion at the Executive Session, Korn dismissed it as consisting of unfounded allegations and rumor. After all, there had been no investigation.

Regaining slight mobility, I interrupted. "What about the inquiry you were supposed to have conducted after our last meeting?"

The dean bristled, then responded by telling me there was a very substantial difference between an "inquiry" and an "investigation." There had been no formal investigation into Gerry's professional behavior where evidence was collected, where those bringing complaints were identified, and certainly not where Gerry had been given the chance to defend himself. In other words, I thought, David Korn had the opportunity to find the evidence he needed but did not bother to even look, and was quite surprised at what surfaced at the Executive Session.

Dean Korn continued. He felt that so much innuendo was now circulating about Gerald Silverberg it could well damage his career. Reopening the search would not solve the problem, no matter what I thought. If Gerry was denied the chair position, it would be as if there had already been an adverse judgment against him, completely without a fair trial. Korn told me he planned to start a formal investigation to explore the allegations I had raised, and until that investigation was complete, Gerry would remain as acting chair of neurosurgery, and the search, which had not been formally closed, would remain in abeyance. Robert Cutler (Senior Associate Dean for Faculty Affairs) and the dean had met with Gerry and a friend of his, also identified as an attorney, the evening before and they had decided on this course of action. While it was agreeable to all of them, Korn told me, Gerry was not very happy about it—not too surprisingly. After taking a deep breath, Korn, in an effort to increase my discomfort, told me bluntly it would have been far preferable for everyone to have been able to handle this whole matter quietly and discreetly.

He glared at me, and I remembered Dave Kuechle's admonition to control my anger, so did not verbalize my thoughts: Sir, without the publicity, Dr. Silverberg would now be chair of my department. I also knew intrusion of legal counsel had been significant in adjusting the dean's thinking and undoubtedly was directing his actions now.

Korn's angry glare suddenly changed into a sarcastic half smile, and, realizing he was now in total control again, told me, gleefully, about the numerous letters he had received since yesterday about how wonderful Gerald Silverberg was. He stood up and twisted his right arm behind his back, with a fake grimace, then abruptly sat down again, placing his elbows on the circular table and holding his head in his hands. He looked at me, absorbing the expression of disbelief on my face, then leisurely leaned back in his chair, extended his frame, hands now behind his head, still watching. The long pause ended. He then said I should take a year of leave to decide what I wanted to do with my life. Korn was not very optimistic I would be able to work at Stanford until a final decision had been reached, and after a year away, thought my options might be more clearly defined. He hesitated, then told me in a rush of words he was leaving town on vacation, would not return until the final week in August, and Robert Cutler would handle "this matter" from now on.

Korn stood up, turned his back to me, walked the few steps to his desk, and picked up a pile of papers, creating an immediate impenetrable but invisible shield between the two of us. The audience was over. My legs and feet felt numb as I shuffled out of his office in total shock. A mere seven days before I had been so very happy. On returning to my office that morning, I had sufficient presence of mind to type out a summary of our discussion.

From start to finish the meeting had been a total disaster. Although I did not know what I would do with the information, at that low point I had an insatiable desire to learn whether a deal had been forged between Gerry and David Korn, information that might explain the dean's uneasiness with his executives' advice, as well as his current change of direction. I phoned Professor Josh Mundle, chair of the Department of Neurobiology, and asked if he had a few minutes to see me. I wanted to reach him before news of the dean's change of plan was announced to his executive group. "Come right on over now," he kindly invited. His office was in an adjacent building.

"Josh, I don't need much of your time. I've only a couple of questions, having to do with Corinne and Morgan. I've heard they're definitely leaving, but can you tell me when Gerry first approached you about housing Morgan in neurosurgery?

His answer was immediate and given without consulting a calendar. He said it had to have been sometime in March or early April. The dean had asked Gerry if he could, thinking neurobiology was close enough to neurosurgery so Morgan's working in a clinical department would not be viewed as a totally absurd idea. I asked if the discussion had included anything about my laboratories at the VA. Josh's memory of the plan was that Morgan was to be given my research space at the VA because Gerry assured them I had no funding. I was startled by what he said, but kept quiet. Gerry had lied. At the time I had both an NIH grant and funding from industry—he had never inquired about my grant support. If I were out of money, Gerry, as acting chair, should have offered me interim financial aid from departmental funds to keep my laboratory going. I had never asked for any because I had no need for any. "Was David Korn involved in any of these discussions?"

It turns out all three of them had been in the office together when details of the plan were finalized—Gerry, David Korn, and Josh Mundle. Gerry's offer had been thoroughly discussed and the dean approved it. Josh also told me there was no question in his mind the dean intended to name Gerry as chair all along, and that Gerry was aware of that plan. Corinne and Morgan had been reassured by both Cutler and Korn not to worry about his acting position—Gerry could appoint and support Morgan without any problem.

Now I knew. Well in advance of my resignation, Dean Korn, in concert with Professor Silverberg, had been actively involved in trying to transfer my VA laboratories to another person without my knowledge or agreement. My research funding had not been important. Gerry and the dean had made a deal—the chair position in exchange for keeping Corinne Spitz. Gerry had upheld his part of the bargain—except he needed my laboratories. So obsessed was he about becoming chair, he was unable to share any credit with me for having saved Corinne. He had not had the decency to ask if I could accommodate Morgan in my research space. As a dictatorial department leader, he thought he could make this unilateral decision without my concurrence, and had done so.

Corinne had told Dean Korn in May she and Morgan were seriously considering the offer from UC Berkeley. Could Stanford match their offer in terms of research space? With Corinne threatening an imminent departure, Korn now could not wait for his neurosurgery chair search committee to generate its final list of candidates, which, with gentle prodding, would have included Gerry as the "best" (and only) inside candidate. He abruptly called off the search, without even informing the search committee, appointed Gerry as permanent chair, and triggered my resignation—a move both he and Gerry fully expected. At that point my resignation was a crucial element for their plan to succeed, and I had not disappointed them. If, instead, I had meekly accepted Gerry's appointment and remained on the faculty, Gerry, as chair, had planned to assign my laboratories to Morgan, or at the very least, require me to share my research space—space I had developed on my own with absolutely no help or funding from the department.

But both Dean Korn and Gerry expected my departure from the faculty would be in May, not September. Once I left, Gerry thought, he could reassign my laboratories to Morgan Idlewild. My delayed termination date meant my group was still working in the space and would continue to occupy it for the next three months. Thus Gerry would be forced to wait until September so he could avoid any appearance of having made a deal. But Morgan and Corinne had to make their employment decision before September, and, indeed, anticipated signing a contract with UC Berkeley during the first part of August. All at once I realized it had been Dean Korn who had directed Gerry to offer my laboratories to Morgan in July immediately before he left on his three-week trip, in a last desperate attempt to keep Corinne Spitz on the faculty. The fact that Gerry did not control my research space was of no concern to the dean, nor did the dean care that I had active grant support. When I resigned in late May, the dean thought he had acquired the necessary research space to complete his scheme formulated two months earlier. It hit me like a fist in the stomach to realize, of necessity, the dean's plan had been predicated all along on my departure from the medical school. Corinne, a good friend of mine, now attuned to the dean's little games, had refused to play. She told me none of the offers from the dean about Morgan's position and space had seemed genuine.

In retrospect, I realized the dean's delay of more than a week between receipt and formal acceptance of my resignation might well have been in response to its September 1 activation date. He would have preferred, and really expected, my immediate departure in May, probably spent the week debating whether he could move up the date, but, for political reasons, knew I was justified in delaying the action, and so let it be. When thinking back to all the numerous embarrassing letters of reference Korn had written for me since 1986 for every conceivable job opening away from Stanford, I also was now aware he had desired and had worked to effect my absence long before 1991.

David Korn has always seemed troubled by me. However, I believe he thought he understood and controlled Professor Corinne Spitz perfectly, and anticipated she would owe him forever for his having saved her career, as well as Morgan's. The dean misjudged Corinne and failed to recognize that Corinne had strength and resolve and was willing to pull up stakes and leave. I think David Korn viewed his few upper-level women faculty as totally naive about the academic political game. They were push-overs. They never instigated revolution and after a bit of whining, and maybe shedding a few tears, they always stayed, regardless of how unfairly they were being treated.

Circumstances beyond his control had prevented Gerry from

rescuing Corinne Spitz for the dean. In good faith, however, he had carried through with his part of the bargain, and, in exchange, he had been promised a chairmanship. Now, with his attorney's help, Gerry had managed to get the dean and himself back on track, and in the past twenty-four hours Gerry had regained his membership in the "good ol' boys' club" and again was the dean's friend and favorite candidate for chair of the department.

By suggesting a year's leave of absence to me, which would be without pay, Korn was responding to the directive from his executives that I be maintained on the faculty. However, he was also recommending I get out of his way, certainly in the short term, but hopefully permanently. Without my being around as a monitor he could conduct whatever type of "investigation" he desired, and finding little or nothing, could justify his choice of Professor Silverberg to the medical community. My "reflective" state away from the medical school would not sustain media interest, and David Korn could finally dismantle that source of extreme irritation and power, the one element he had not anticipated when he had formulated his plan. Everything would be neatly in place, on the dean's terms, for me to accept or reject upon my return after a year of contemplation.

The next day Ken Bloem called to tell me I was no longer being considered for the Chief of Staff position. Over the phone his voice carried embarrassment; he gave no reasons for the decision, and I did not ask for any, feeling confident I already knew. David Korn was batting 1.000. I called Sally Hawthorne at the EEOC and told her I would work with the commission in their attempt to obtain information about Stanford University and its employment practices during my last month at the medical school. It was obvious there was no place for me at this institution and I began in earnest to obliterate an academic career from my office. As large boxes of junk to be thrown away accumulated, the secretaries at the VA began talking about a "farewell" dinner for me, unknowingly adding yards to my shroud of negativity and despair. I had just over three more weeks of employment before I would leave and start a new life.

I reached Dave Kuechle at Harvard and brought him up to date. I asked him for his thoughts. After a long pause his answer was, "I think you've just lost." I do not remember ever in my life feeling so desolate, so alone, and so absolutely pounded by the power and force of institutional strength.

9 I was plunged into a black hole of immobilizing depression, which became my constant companion. To deal with the stress in my professional life I have always found comfort in my "church"—a daily run in the hills, with trees, meadows, and patterns of filtered morning sun and shade, watching my dog go bananas in her doggy world of horse manure and squirrels. The religious experience covers all seasons: tiny, ethereal wildflowers—pink, bright light blue, white, and yellow—in early spring, giving way to beautiful bunches of wild iris, ranging in color from snow white to the deepest of royal purples; the warm, day-old air along the trails in summer, mixing at the top with cool swirls of fog born at the ocean; the lush, soft running carpet of dead leaves in autumn; and the rebirth of it all brought by winter rains, turning the dirt trails to mud and my white and black-spotted dog to brown. God is there every morning.

But now my run in the emerging daylight would be interrupted by the sudden onset of unwelcome breathless sobs and flooding tears, forcing me to walk for short distances. Morning after morning, there was no peace and I found no pleasure in the beauty of the forested hills. I could not sleep past three in the morning, and spent the two hours before dawn and the alarm awake and restless, thinking about what had happened and what the future would bring. This was not a game I would win, not as an individual pitted against the institutional power I had confronted. Events had sucked me into an abyss, and I saw no easy escape from its depths—the steps I had taken could not be retraced or erased. The students had been correct—this dean had no intention of working to change the sexist culture of our medical school (except, perhaps, superficially for the benefit of the press). Dejectedly, I realized Korn had never tried to persuade me that my stance taken on account of Gerry's behavior was wrong—to him, it was just unimportant. Gerry's conduct, past and present, was inconsequential. There were too many others like him. Korn would be harshly criticized within our community were he to use Gerry as an isolated example. Korn abhorred criticism. Furthermore, my using the press to open the imperfections of our work and study environment for the entire world to see and critique was a serious transgression. Untrustworthy and devious were adjectives that the dean would now add to my string of personality flaws. More than ever, for his own peace of mind, Dean David Korn had to assure my departure would be September 1.

I also had doubts about what I had done. The press had carried the whole situation much farther than I had ever intended or could have imagined. A true sense of conventional outrage had never overwhelmed me. Gerry's conduct, as well as that of others, while troublesome, had never been intolerable. Aggravating, maddening, belittling, but not limiting, in any true sense, until my laboratories had been given away. Insiders shrugged and said this was all part of the academic environment, an ongoing, ever-present fierce competition for ultimate control of resources. It could have happened to anyone in this survival-of-the-fittest game. Yet, in stark contrast, those on the outside looking in told me my world was awful, despicable, tragic, and, yes, outrageous. But it was a world I had accepted, and one I had never questioned. Did I have the right suddenly to turn 180 degrees in the opposite direction, hurling invectives at where I had been? The only true outrage I felt was toward the dean for his misguided decision and dishonesty about stopping the search in the first place and his current intent to conduct a "formal" investigation. He was just buying time until I left so he would be unobstructed in crowning his personal choice for chair.

Senior Associate Dean for Faculty Affairs Dr. Robert Cutler called late in the morning three days after my disastrous meeting with Dean Korn. His soft, throaty voice was matter-of-fact, the call informational. Cutler had been assigned the task of holding investigative hearings about Gerry and had decided on the format for those hearings. He told me he planned to convene a panel before I left in September, but sincerely doubted the investigative process could be completed by that time.

Robert Cutler, M.D., is a neurologist by training and became Associate Dean for Faculty shortly after David Korn was appointed dean of the medical school in 1984. The "Senior" was added to his title in 1988. Professor Cutler had been saved from a nasty interpersonal problem within his department by the offer of a position in the dean's office, and I believe Bob has been eternally grateful to David Korn for the rescue. Certainly no dean could have asked for a more loyal and steadfast partner over the years. I have known Cutler since I joined the faculty in 1975, a year after he did, and we have always enjoyed a decent working relationship. He had ended a note to me about my resignation with "As I hope you know, Frances, I deeply regret your decision to leave the faculty." I had no reason to question his sincerity.

The investigative panel would hear from anyone who wished to appear before it. However, all those willing to share information had to agree, in advance, to have the proceedings taped and typed into a transcript. Subsequently, the entire unedited transcript would be given to Gerry, with full disclosure of the person's identity. While the intent was to provide him with due process, Gerry would also know just who had appeared, as well as the totality of what had been said in an informal setting. In the future, were he named chair, he would know exactly with whom to get even. It was an orchestrated format to uncover no evidence whatever. However, I was surprised by how rapidly Bob Cutler apparently was responding to Dean Korn's directive and had grim satisfaction in knowing the executive group had forced the two of them to struggle, for a couple of weeks at least, with the possibility of aberrant professional behavior by Professor Silverberg.

Bob also asked if I thought Gerry should remain on the faculty if some of the "worrisome material" could, indeed, be proven. I found his question quite troubling. While it would send a clear and unambiguous message to our community about proper conduct, dismissing one sexist, arrogant faculty surgeon would not change the basic culture of the medical school—not with David Korn as its dean. I told Bob Cutler I saw no reason a highly trained, skilled neurosurgeon and teacher should be discharged from the faculty for behavior many were guilty of—"but just because you decide to keep him, doesn't mean he should be made chair—stop trying to put him on a pedestal!"

Dean Cutler's next comment told me he had missed the point I had tried to make. He told me he would need my help. I replied that in the time I had left, I would be more than willing to meet with his panel, even under what I considered adverse conditions. Also, wishing to disown any appearance of covert activity, I casually informed Bob that the EEOC had been in contact, "in case you think the legal office should know." His voice over the phone did not relay any apprehension or concern over my news.

At the beginning of the second week in August, I met with Sally Hawthorne from the EEOC. Ms. Hawthorne was younger than I had expected and visibly pregnant. I asked when her baby was due. "In another month—I'll be going on maternity leave in a couple of weeks." She added, "Apropos of your experiences, when I first put on maternity clothes, my colleagues suddenly treated me as if I could no longer think, that my brain had gone to my belly." She laughed. "Now I put up with men patting my stomach, as if I were a Buddha and they were getting something magical from it. When you're pregnant the universe suddenly owns you, and, 'poor dear,' we know your mind is occupied elsewhere." She laughed again, able to enjoy the humor of her situation, which, after all, was temporary.

In order for Sally Hawthorne to file a class action lawsuit she needed discrete episodes of discrimination which could be verified by willing witnesses. Her investigators were encountering employees who were reluctant to talk to them, even after they themselves had initially approached the commission. The fear of retribution and job loss, and, for female physicians, career truncation, was for many too high a price to pay. Staff and nontenured faculty had no occupational security at Stanford. A female doctor from the Radiology Department had contacted the EEOC office but, without tenure, had been reluctant to follow through with a formal complaint. She told me, after her brief encounter with the commission, she intuitively discerned that academic medical centers and universities had a degree of informal immunity not shared with other workplaces, and might well not be subject to the same degree of scrutiny as a law firm or a business. However, to help Sally Hawthorne make a decision about whether Stanford was guilty of unfair practices, I agreed to meet with the EEOC attorney assigned to the case, and, in the last three weeks of August, help the commission obtain information by persuading women to share their employment experiences.

Coincident with David Korn's efforts to assure my departure from the faculty, two legal briefs had been sent to me as informational items by two women academicians, both physicians, one at Albert Einstein Medical School and the other at the NIH. Because of parallels to my situation, reading them was fascinating, although depressing. I learned that the institutional response to threat was quite stereotyped. Sexual harassment and discrimination based on gender frequently had little or nothing to do with sexuality and everything to do with power and control—especially over a professional woman's career. Clearly, I was not alone.

Both women had excellent credentials at their respective institutions. As they established their academic reputations and became increasingly competitive, they had apparently threatened male physicians in their respective departments. The knee-jerk response by those threatened was to eliminate the two women, one by denying her a third-year fellowship position, the other by labeling her a "troublemaker." Neither woman had tenure. The troublemaker, internationally recognized in her field, discovered that a chapter she had written and published previously listed her boss as the sole author when it was republished—her name was gone. She obtained a court order to stop him from distributing her work as his. Thus the misdeed was revealed to the public at large, embarrassing the institution. Her efforts to regain the rights to her work were rewarded by being escorted from her office by a security guard and having her keys forcibly taken from her. She sued her boss for copyright infringement. Subsequently, the plagiarizer was promoted. In the other woman's case, when she objected to a display of demeaning sexist cards and cartoons, as well as to personal derogatory verbal comments from her boss, she found herself ostracized from the main research group, had plum assignments taken from her, saw her research published by others, and then had her academic career assassinated by being forced to leave her fellowship during her last year. Both women were engaged in legal battles, claiming gender discrimination and unfair termination. Although early court decisions supported them, they had huge debts from legal fees. Neither could find employment. For them, legal action would not resurrect the professional lives they had once envisioned for themselves.

Interestingly, during the more than two months since my resignation, I had been criticized by some as not being representative of the class of women (and minorities) who really needed help. It is true that with tenure my job had been protected. Those in unprotected job situations, or students, were the usual favored prey for those with power. In order to avoid becoming part of the food chain, women physicians in the academy generally learn to walk a narrow precipice called "compromise," knowing they will be judged as never doing anything quite good enough, yet at the same time realizing they dare not excel and draw attention to themselves. My neurosurgical colleagues rarely forget my mistakes, but my greater sin is to do a difficult surgical case well. In reviewing promotion papers for a female assistant professor at an Advisory Board meeting, one of my male colleagues on the board, with a touch of humor, introduced the candidate with "She probably isn't as good as these papers and letters suggest, but she's still pretty good." Her academic performance was one all of us would have been proud to own.

Saturday morning I went to my office to continue the miserable process of incrementally winding down my career by throwing out files. It was remarkable how many reports, memos, and letters I had accumulated. It was equally remarkable how most of the information was no longer useful or pertinent. I opened files I had not seen for years. They brought back memories of committees, discussions, searches for an athletic director and a football coach. For brief moments people from the past came alive, ghosts of good cheer and happier times. It would have been less brutal, less traumatic to have thrown the files away without regard for their contents. But somehow I needed to remember; I had forgotten so much of the joy I once experienced in my academic life.

The brief discussion on the phone with Bob Cutler remained in the back of my mind. It was like a toothache—tolerable but unpleasant. As a relief from cleaning chores, I tried once more, and wrote a letter to Cutler on the computer, the floor at my feet cluttered with papers, boxes, files, and journals.

I wrote about the world women doctors inhabited at the medical center. It was one full of dichotomies—we were regarded as a competent physician by our patients, but were a "honey" or "sweetie" to our peers; we respected certain of our colleagues for their professional capabilities, knowing, at the same time, that some of their behavior was reprehensible. I thought that most women were willing to continue a dichotomous existence *if* the gulf did not widen and *if* there was tangible evidence of commitment to evolutionary change by our leaders, leading to a reduction in the dichotomy. The increasing number of women entering medicine demanded it. I told Bob his "investigation" was unlikely to yield the data he needed. Gerry's sexist behavior would be impossible to quantify (as no one else's behavior had ever been investigated) and would disturb some but not others. I wrote, "For twenty-three years I productively worked *with* him; I cannot work *for* him because his demeaning behavior to me and others is an insult and an embarrassment to that department of which I was a member. . . . Remember, I have not 'charged' Dr. Silverberg with anything except being an improper choice on the part of the dean for chair, Department of Neurosurgery." By the time I finished writing the letter, ending with "I leave this, my second home, with a great deal of sorrow and unfulfilled dreams, but remain ever hopeful that eventually, that which is right shall prevail," tears were streaming down my face.

Robert Cutler dictated a rapid response focused entirely on "the investigation" and ignored the fact that subtleties are the heart of the much broader harassment/free speech debate. He concentrated, instead, on discrete, measurable charges. Grimly, I realized Deans Korn and Cutler had chosen to interpret my published opinion piece very concretely. To them my written editorial, in and of itself, was sufficient to have lodged specific charges against Gerry which could be proven either true or false. With that interpretation they had the right and duty to investigate those charges, and I told Bob, without any hesitation, I looked forward to meeting with his investigative panel to tell them about the world of neurosurgery at Stanford Medical School. Retribution from Gerry was of no concern to me; I would be gone. However, I had considerable doubt others would be willing to help Cutler with his fact-finding mission, given that every contributed detail would be revealed to Gerry.

As had become routine, I sent copies of both my memo to Cutler and his to me to attorney John Tyndall. John had been informed about Korn's involvement in attempting to reassign my laboratories. This action had profound legal implications, as it could be interpreted as unequivocal gender discrimination—deliberate intent to limit my professional resources when those of my male colleagues had been left untouched. The neurosurgery laboratories at Stanford were being used by one of the two assistant professors in the department, and no attempt had been made to assign any portion of them to Morgan Idlewild.

John Tyndall was concerned about my participation in the investigative process, as he understood it. He encouraged me to meet with the panel, if invited, but warned me not to solicit evidence from others. "If you've asked anyone to appear, they'll have no credibility." For this and other reasons, he thought it time he made his presence known in a nonconfrontational but decisive manner. "Let them know you have legal counsel and are prepared to use it." I concurred with John's thinking—I had nothing to lose by telling the deans an attorney was available to me. John wrote a letter to Senior Associate Dean Cutler, reminding him he had successfully represented me in past legal action and discussed the inadvisability of my "active participation" in the investigation. Instead, he enclosed copies of all the letters I had received since my resignation documenting Gerry's behavior. Tyndall's letter concluded, "I believe my forwarding [the letters] to you breaches no one's sense of privacy or confidence. I trust that they will be treated accordingly and used only for the investigation now being conducted by your office."

The packet contained thirty-seven letters from patients, nurses, and colleagues about episodes of sexist behavior and sexual harassment they had witnessed or experienced in relation to Gerry. Some of these had been sent to David Korn, either directly or by "cc." I had no idea whether Korn had shared these with Bob Cutler. At any rate, Bob Cutler now knew what I knew and also knew all the letters were in the hands of my attorney.

Phil and I became quite reflective. He was still hoping for a miracle despite my last awful meeting with the dean. He recognized tremendous ambivalence in my thinking about decisions for the future. How could I give up my career at Stanford when I had devoted my entire life to it? Yet how could I continue to work with Gerry as acting chair where I could not be fully functional? His verbal abuse would continue unabated, intensified and magnified because I had dared to challenge him and his absolute power. But there were issues larger than my personal ones. What did my departure say about a medical school and university that had, after all, extended an extraordinary level of opportunity and support to me for most of my life? Did I owe anything to that institution?

Mental peace had been elusive since early June. Every half mile I ran in the early morning felt like a very long mile. Running through the smell of dry warm redwoods and the pungency of wet sunburnt meadow grass, I did considerable serious, contemplative thinking those early August mornings, and gradually expanded a narrow focus into a broader one.

My conflict was not about Professor Gerald Silverberg and the chair position, but about a medical culture that condoned stereotypic thinking, outdated behavior, and an arrogant superiorist ideology coupled with stubborn resistance to change. A culture shift was essential for women because of the negative, limiting impact of the status quo on our careers. But harassment was an embarrassing consideration for men. Why was there any question over a man's *right* to flirt with women? It was a time-honored interplay between the sexes and both men and women enjoyed it—or at least acted as if they did. So why were men suddenly castigated for conduct that had always unequivocally defined their God-given male-superior status in the medical environment? Many men were quite angry with me for having brought the issue into the open, feeling I had driven an unnecessary wedge between them and their female friends and colleagues. A number made a point of telling me, "Gee, now I don't dare meet with a girl (sic) in my office by myself." And "there's no way I'd ever mentor a woman, not with all the talk and gossip around this place." While a generalized condemnation of my male peer group was totally unfair, I listened to this type of comment with considerable suspicion. Yet I certainly knew that there were good people at Stanford, many of them, whose professional and personal behavior was beyond reproach, and almost all of them in my physician peer group happened to be men.

Regardless of her field, every woman practicing medicine today does owe a portion of her career to men, and a few women, who were willing to teach her, sponsor her, cheer for her, and guide her. A mentoring role should be so natural for a physician, and a mentor relationship is one important rung on a career ladder, providing contacts, inside information, advice about grants, publications, career advancement, and other intangible aids to success. Mentors for my generation of academic women doctors were men, when they could be found. A true mentor sincerely and genuinely works to forge, build, and solidify the career of another, without need to augment his or her own status through the work of those being mentored. With same-gender mentorships, marvelous nonthreatening intimacy between two people can develop, evolving into a lifelong partnership of having shared something very special. Unfortunately, a close mentor relation between a man and a woman, especially if the woman is younger and the one being mentored, is often fragile, as societal assumptions work to turn the relationship into something it is not. Mixed-gender mentorships must be carefully designed and often consist of a delicate balance of distance between two people. Too often the societal perception is correct, as I learned at one of our infrequent women's faculty meetings. We had broken into small groups to talk about mentors and how we might improve the process for us. One of my group began rhapsodizing about what a marvelous, wonderful, somewhat older mentor she had found early in her career, and how he continued to support and help her today, even though they were no longer at the same institution. The rest of us were enviously fascinated, and I tentatively asked how the relationship had initially developed. What was the secret behind her successful coup? Without any embarrassment whatever, she answered, "Oh, we had a long-term affair—he has four children and a wife who didn't understand him, and I was able to give him a connection he really needed." She was totally oblivious to the obvious abuse of power their relationship represented. Thus, while young men take a mentor relation almost as a birthright, many, if not most, women physicians lack access to an appropriate mentor, a phenomenon that can severely handicap her career.

As I looked back, I felt deep gratitude to many who had helped mold my career, enthusiastically, genuinely, without a power play or ulterior motive. Besides Dr. Hanbery, there was the neuroradiologist who taught me the art of cerebral arteriography. A beloved orthopedic surgeon, now deceased, who showed me, hands-on and with infinite patience, the intricacies of spinal fusion technique and what bones could and would not do. An idiosyncratic neuropathologist, world-renowned, had constructed, block by block, a sturdy foundation for my future research program. Even though, long ago, I had rejected their specialty, there were plastic surgeons who avidly supported my career and made me feel good about myself and my choice. Over the years there were numerous anesthesiologists whose talent and compassion made difficult cases less difficult and, more important, provided a buffer between misogynistic surgeons and me, telling the former, and sometimes the latter, without compunction, "You're really full of it!" Two previous chairs of the Department of Surgery, still on the faculty, were still members of my booster club. And so many of my male neurosurgery peers outside of Stanford who, at the time I resigned, wrote to offer condolences, bravos, jobs, and instant, unquestioned support.

What was my obligation, if any, to this bizarre world of medicine where abuse and compassion coexisted and were not infrequently delivered by the same individual? Had I unearthed an astonishing opportunity to confront tradition and tacit assumptions, and in so doing change an entire culture by affecting individual behavior? Or had I been an outsider, a foreigner, all along, deceiving myself into believing I really belonged? Maybe it was my destiny to dwell forever on the fringe, not ever being in a position to change anything about my professional life or the lives of others. By leaving I would never know.

I talked with many friends at the university, for the most part not at the medical school. Professor Jeff Pfeffer indignantly told me, "You've just started the fight, you can't quit now." Recognizing that an investigation was only a promise (the panel had not been activated, despite Bob Cutler's articulated intent) and any tangible action by Dean Korn lay in the future, a member of the Advisory Board recommended I capitalize on these minuscule concessions in order to thwart the enemy. His advice? "Grin like a Cheshire cat, tell them they're great, and come back!"

I was so hungry for peace in my life, away from the press, away from unending hostility and animosity. To stay meant more of the same, day by grueling day, with no guarantee of future happiness. I needed more time. By departing on September 1 I would leave Dean Korn without a vestige of guilt or remorse over my scuttled professional life, and I knew, despite all his frenetic activity devoted to establishing committees and focus groups, with our present leadership nothing in our culture would change.

On August 28, Phil and I went out to dinner, and in the long evening of sunlight, on the way home, returned to my almost empty office at the VA as if drawn there by a magnet. We sat and stared at each other for many long moments, then decided it was worth doing, if for no other reason than the shock value. We had spent the best years of our lives working for a tenured professoriate—maybe it was time to make tenure work for us. Together we composed a letter on the computer to Dean Cutler:

Dear Bob:

After our last conversation a couple of weeks ago I have sought the counsel of many members of the academic community both at the medical school and within the university. These individuals have persuaded me that David's and your actions to date are sufficiently reassuring of your commitment to taking appropriate action with regard to the question of leadership for the Department of Neurosurgery that it is in my best interest, and in the best interest of Stanford University, to withdraw my resignation from the institution and return to my duties at the Veterans Affairs Medical Center and at the medical school. If, as David Korn has told me, I am "unable to work at Stanford" I will use my one-eighth time [there] to work on a project with two colleagues in the School of Education. I have been advised that a leave of absence creates too many unacceptable possibilities.

I signed the letter "Fran" and copied Dean Korn and Gerry Silverberg. I also sent a blind copy to President Donald Kennedy, letting him know the letter had been distributed the evening of August 28. On our way home Phil and I delivered the original and one copy to the locked dean's office, pushing them under the door. We put Gerry's copy in his office mailbox.

I knew Dean Korn had no real choice but to accept the rescinding. The media were still interested in resolution of the story, and he had told them numerous times, awash with hypocritical tears, how much he regretted my resignation and how enthusiastically he would welcome my return to the faculty. He was to get his wish. Now that I knew the identity of my real enemy, I was making the decision to stay and fight an all-out war. Like a snake shedding its skin, I discarded any residual victim mentality and went on the offensive. The time had come to hold David Korn accountable for his behavior toward others. The battle for equal opportunity for women in our workplace would be fought over Gerald Silverberg's professional decorum, but if my allegations about his behavior were formally substantiated, David Korn, along with many others, would be found just as guilty.

Robert Cutler wrote a gracious note the next morning which was delivered to the VA by messenger.

> *Dear Fran:*
>
> *I want you to know how very pleased I was to find your letter of 28 August under the door early this morning. In fact, I called my wife to inform her of the news! From an administrative point of view, your earlier notice of intent to resign on August 31, 1991, has been withdrawn.*
>
> *If there prove to be difficult times ahead and you believe I can be helpful as a mediator, I hope you will call on me. I will offer the same to Gerry.*
>
> *I look forward to our continuing as colleagues.*
>
> *Sincerely,*
> *Robert W. P. Cutler*

He had copied President Kennedy and the university provost. Cutler decided to face the press after the Labor Day weekend and asked the public relations office to prepare a release for September 4.

The press release was given to the media late in the afternoon. The next day all of the local papers, as well as *The New York Times* and *The Washington Post,* carried the story, relying on an overly positive statement drawn up by the university. In it, "Cutler confirmed that Vice President and Dean David Korn has appointed a committee to review some of the issues Dr. Conley has raised and that a decision concerning the permanent leadership of the neurosurgery department will be influenced by the outcome of the committee's deliberations. . . . Conley said she was surprised by the reaction to her article and the media blitz and international attention she was subjected to afterward, but she has no regrets because 'the message got out.' "

The media barrage was back with full intensity. Rita was handling phone calls like a seasoned native. This time I avoided a media circus at the VA; Cutler and I faced the press together in a room at the medical school.

A few minutes before, I met Bob in his office. We hugged each other spontaneously, and my eyes filled with tears. "It's been a rough three months," I said. Bob offered me a box of Kleenex. Composure regained, I continued, "I'll be as positive as I can, but I'm not going to lie."

Cutler said he did not expect me to—I should try to keep things as general as possible. I think he understood my ambivalence about returning. He was also concerned about what I might say.

He put on a freshly starched white laboratory coat, and as we opened the door to leave his office, I said, "You know, Bob, what David did with my labs was wrong."

Bob answered that he knew—and that it should never have happened. This was the first indication I had that he was aware of past events and probably had some understanding about the potential legal implications. He did not mention having received the packet of letters from my attorney.

Television, radio, and print media folk who had gathered in the amphitheater-style classroom were clustered in the bottom rows of padded folding seats. Standing at the lectern area looking up at people and cameras, Dean Cutler and I answered questions for about twenty minutes. I did most of the talking until questions were asked about the various committees and focus groups commissioned to explore the climate at our medical school. Bob answered these. In my statements I tried to put a positive slant on the school and its dean and how they were responding to the issues I had raised. I confess it made me feel more than a little hypocritical, because I knew in fact nothing had changed. I had met many of the reporters before, and could detect skepticism in their questions and the way they asked them. They simply did not believe the school had revised its attitudes so rapidly about sexism and sexual harassment. They were wondering who and what were driving me—what was the hidden agenda I had agreed to, and why? I was quite adamant that I was not returning to my former work conditions, and never would. After all, an investigation was now being conducted. Depending on its outcome, I might still leave, but at least an effort was being made to obtain information about my allegations. I am not sure how much I believed about what I was saying. That evening, Phil, who had seen the television coverage, said I had been "much too kind."

On September 11, I received a brief, chilly note from Gerry, the first communication from him since his letter acknowledging, with "sadness," my resignation.

Dear Dr. Conley:

The dean has informed me that you have asked him to rescind your resignation and he has agreed to do it. I am not sure what your plans are and how you wish to be reintegrated with the department. I would be happy to meet with you to go over your ideas and will accommodate your schedule as much as I can. Please call to arrange an appointment as soon as possible. [A second paragraph informed me that the VA residency program in neurosurgery would likely be closed in the next year, meaning I would be left alone at

*the VA without a resident or other faculty, and be required
to take call there every night and weekend.]*
                           Sincerely, Gerald D. Silverberg, M.D.

The letter was signed with a full signature and was copied to
David Korn and Robert Cutler. I was not surprised by its frigid
formality. It certainly indicated tense times lay ahead. So I accepted Bob Cutler's offer to act as a mediator between Gerry and
me. Our three calendars did not match until the first week in
October.

When Phil saw Gerry's letter that evening, he wrote across it,
"the start of Gerry's chicken-shit responses," then copied it and
sent it to his group of friends who were interested in our continuing saga. The neurosurgical service at the Palo Alto VA has
weathered the storm although it was threatened a few more times.

The media coverage of my return unleashed another flood of
letters. The *Los Angeles Times* asked me to write a follow-up
editorial for them, which I did. It was published under their
choice of title: "Why I'm Going Back to Stanford: I Am Not a
Lonely Victim" (*Los Angeles Times*, September 15, 1991). I
would never have chosen "victim." A "victim" has no power to
act, to speak, to write, or to effect change.

Finally the identities of those serving on a panel of inquiry
were announced. Dean Cutler was chairing it. He was joined by
a professor of urology, a psychologist, and the director of nursing,
representing the hospital.

I had known Dr. Davis Grant since medical school days. He
is charming, decent, and a rare and welcome antithesis to the
surgeon stereotype. He had always treated me with kindness and
respect. Davis was a regular attendee at the infamous Thursday
surgical departmental luncheons, and would laugh with the rest
until the humor disintegrated into true debauchery and became
directed at a defenseless target, usually junior faculty and/or a
woman. Then he would blush deeply with embarrassment. I knew
he could graphically depict the inner world of surgery at Stanford

Medical School for his fellow panelists, and would find no need to embellish the description with editorial comment.

Alison Stone, Ph.D., and I had worked together on a couple of committees and I knew her to be fair, honest, and insightful. But I feared she would also be easily swayed by the dominant members of the panel. She was someone who would build and support consensus at almost any cost.

I did not know Susan Flint-Hubbell, R.N., well. However, because she was a high-ranking hospital administrator and not a faculty member, her presence on the panel signaled a serious intent to explore the totality of our work world—the clinics and hospital as well as the medical school. In addition, hospital employees who might agree to meet with the panel would feel more comfortable doing so because of her presence. Despite the delay in convening the panel, I became convinced Bob Cutler would undertake a thorough and honest investigation, and wondered if my return to the faculty had fueled his dedication to the task.

Stanford University starts its school year late in comparison with many institutions of higher education. I worried that returning students would feel betrayed by my decision. Had I somehow given up and relinquished their cause by crawling back? While they had witnessed flames scorch my running shoes when they left in June, most believed only my charred remnants would remain upon their return at the end of September. How welcome, or credible, is a resurrected rabble-rouser?

Ushering in the new academic year, the orientation issue of the *Stanford Daily*, the student-run newspaper, ran a picture and story about my "return" to campus. Medical students had been interviewed for the article and some were "hopeful" and others "not confident at all" the culture at the medical school would improve, given all the committees and focus groups formed by the dean. The two grievances filed against Mark Perlroth had literally disappeared without any announced resolution—the students had heard nothing and were convinced they never would. As for me, I had "done the right thing" in coming back, according to the student reporters.

The September 16 issue of *U.S. News & World Report*, in its regular feature entitled "People," covered the withdrawal of my resignation in a small paragraph accompanied by my picture. One of the in-depth articles contained in that issue and heralded on the front cover was "The Brief on Clarence Thomas."

10 In early October, Drs. Cutler, Silverberg, and Conley met face to face for about twenty minutes. I had been extremely apprehensive about the meeting, and Bob Cutler also seemed uncomfortable. Gerry was encased in a cool rage. Little was accomplished in repairing the rift. I told Gerry so long as the investigation was being conducted I could not imagine working at Stanford Medical Center and would continue duties only at the VA. In exchange for not seeing patients at Stanford or taking weekend call there, I would not participate in any departmental distribution payment at the end of the year (such payments can be sizable for our faculty, as our billings are high relative to other medical disciplines). Gerry directed his comments exclusively to Dean Cutler, as if I were not present. He seemed relieved I would not interfere with his world and was quite nonchalant, almost insolent, about the investigation which was underway.

I met with Cutler's investigative panel on October 10 for ninety minutes in the dean's conference room. The conversation was taped. Prior to my interview, the panel had talked with a few others, although I was not privy to their identity or the content of the discussion. Except for a few questions about how loose Gerry was with his hands around women and inquiries into alleged racist behavior and comments, the focus was his suitability for executive leadership.

I relayed the history of my dysfunctional department, going back in time to Dr. Hanbery's tenure and the episode of embezzlement. I shared my views about how difficult it was to be a professional amid a constant barrage of verbal insults and belittling comments that defined my position within my work environment. Even though the comments were not necessarily made in my presence, I knew what was being said—gossip was alive and well in neurosurgery, and Gerry knew his remarks would make the rounds. Deferential and apologetic over the sins of others, Davis Grant, in so many words, told me and the panel he knew exactly what I was talking about—and was sorry.

Prior to this session, I had not thought about whether Gerry was a racist. Racist comments obviously had been relayed by others who preceded me in talking to the panel. I knew Gerry hated Arabs with a vengeance and on rounds, immediately outside of a patient's room, would delight in making uninhibited, scurrilous comments about "camel drivers" and their purported worth to the world. Nevertheless, despite his personal feelings, Gerry operated on many patients from the Middle East, and I never saw him provide them anything but the very best of care.

Susan Flint-Hubbell asked about the nursing staff on our floor at Stanford Hospital and its interaction with Gerry. I said, "I know there are many nurses who are repulsed by his sexist behavior, as well as his inappropriate comments about the basic inferiority of Hispanic nurses or those from the Philippines. I believe many have grave reservations about Gerry being chair of neurosurgery and I think most would dearly love to see someone else appointed. But some of them are very shy and I'm not sure they'll talk, given the way this panel is being run. Gerry'll get even with them."

It had been a cathartic session, in the company of compassionate listeners who were interested in hearing about the broad ramifications of Gerry's behavior within our medical center. The panel was apparently serious about their assignment. At the end I thanked them for being willing to spend their precious time on behalf of my ailing department.

In another part of the country at approximately the same time, a black female law professor from Oklahoma named Anita Hill alleged that Judge Clarence Thomas, President Bush's nominee for the Supreme Court, had sexually harassed her ten years before. The Judiciary Committee and Congress began scrambling, back-pedaling, denying, scrutinizing, and negotiating, all in pursuit of damage control over what was already a highly controversial appointment.

The weekend after I met with the panel, our country and the world were treated to an embarrassing debacle of riveting proportion as the all-male, all-white U.S. Senate Judiciary Committee conducted hearings into alleged harassment by a black man who wished to be a Supreme Court Justice. Phil concentrated all of his waking hours on the TV coverage, and, when the hearings concluded, changed his voting registration from Republican to California's version of "independent"—that is, "decline to state."

Poor Stanford. Just when media interest in my activities was rapidly disappearing, the press returned. I called the head of the News Bureau and asked if I should continue working with the various reporters. The answer: "Oh my yes; we don't want any to accuse us of quashing you." So my considered opinions about the Hill-Thomas event appeared in newspapers, magazines, on radio and TV. *People* magazine even agreed to allow me editorial privilege over an interview they would do; with that promise, I broke my long-standing boycott. Issues raised by the Hill-Thomas confrontation remained newsworthy for a prolonged time. No question their drama extended my fifteen minutes of fame.

I imagine Dr. Gerald Silverberg identified with Judge Clarence Thomas. Neither of them ever expected to have his professional behavior questioned, at least not in a public forum. Both had been blindsided by women, by changing moral standards, and by profound demographic shifts and attention to issues of diversity in the workplace. Neither could have anticipated such rapid truncation of "business as usual," and both, like me, had been oblivious to the undercurrent of discontent spreading like a virus, without regard for occupation or class, within the ranks of working women.

After I returned to my faculty position, my VA office became a place where troubles could be shared. Many people in this country believe publicity—any publicity—means credibility as well as expertise. It was as if my yet unfinished crusade had endowed me with a special form of magic for instantaneous problem solving. Two or three times a week I would receive a phone call or a visit from a woman with a story. Many accounts were long and complicated, most of them compelling and disheartening. I remember one of the first stories in vivid, poignant, gut-wrenching detail.

During the autumn quarter I received a midmorning phone call from a female medical student at Stanford. She asked if I had time to meet with her. "Of course, my office, this afternoon?" She would be there. I knew Sonja, as she had spent time as a clinical clerk on the neurosurgical service at Stanford the year before. She was a good student.

Sonja has a faint accent reflecting her birth and early upbringing in Eastern Europe. Her undergraduate degree is in engineering and she had worked a few years as an engineer before realizing she desired more people contact in her career and returned to school to study medicine. She was tense, almost shaky, as she sat down stiffly in the chair I offered. Leaning forward, she said, "I'm not sure how to begin, but I need some help and advice."

"Start where you want—what's happened?"

"I'm not going to get the residency I want."

"In neurosurgery? I hadn't realized you'd applied."

"No, no, no—not neurosurgery, I want to go into ophthalmology. I haven't received a single interview invitation from any of the programs I applied to—they've ruined me." As she raised her head to look at me, I could see the tears start. Stanford medical students do not all get their first choice of residency, and there are always one or two who do not match in the spring draw; but it is virtually unheard of to be offered no interviews whatever. It was an ugly story.

Sonja began, "I was accepted at other medical schools but chose Stanford because I wanted an academic career—I've been out in the world already and I'm pretty directed. I knew research experience was real important, so as soon as I got here my first year, I went to talk to Dr. Duane Morris here in ophthalmology—my engineering background is a good fit with his work. You know Dr. Morris?" she asked me.

"Yeah, sure, I know who he is." Duane Morris was a Ph.D. researcher at the medical school, internationally known for his work, and had excellent, uninterrupted funding. I suspected his work was responsible for keeping the Department of Ophthalmology in the black.

Sonja continued. "He runs the only research lab in the department, and I asked if I could join it because I really wanted to work on eyes. He was very nice and found a place for me and even found a small stipend, which really helped. I didn't see him again for a couple of months—I was assigned to work with one of the postdocs, so he was directing my project. One afternoon late that first quarter I was working in the lab, and Dr. Morris came up to me, and kind of out of the blue asked if I wanted to go to the opera with him—he said his wife and daughter would go with us. He gave me a date, and I told him I'd need to check with Carl—he's my steady boyfriend. Well, when I got home at night, the two of us talked it over. I don't know, I felt a little funny about it . . ."

"Do others from the lab go to the opera with him?"

Sonja shrugged. "I have no idea, and certainly didn't then."

She paused briefly. "After talking with Carl we decided it was a nice, friendly gesture—you know, it would be a chance for me to get to know him better, and his wife and daughter would be there. I found Dr. Morris the next day and told him I was free on that evening and I'd love to go. He asked if I minded driving to his house. All of us would leave in one car from there. I told him that'd be fine, and he gave me his address and directions how to get there."

Sonja sighed deeply, then continued. "That evening, which was a week or so after I'd last seen him, I drove to his house. He has a circular driveway off the street, and I parked in the front—I didn't see any other car. He met me at the front door, saying that his wife and daughter had decided to stay in Carmel for the evening, so it was just the two of us for the opera. And would I mind driving? I wish I had my life to live over—I should've left right then and told him I'd take a rain check."

Somehow, I knew what was coming. I also knew there was no decision Sonja could have made that evening that would have worked out well. She had already been trapped.

Sonja forced herself to continue her story. "What could I do? We got in my car and I drove to San Francisco. He didn't even have opera tickets!" Sonja forced a sarcastic laugh. "When we got there he bought standing-room tickets and spent the first act brushing up against me, kept asking me to take my coat off. It was real warm, but I kept my coat on. At intermission, thank God, we ran into a couple, friends of his, and after talking a bit, the wife suggested I sit with her for the rest of the opera and let the two men stand."

I interrupted. "Any reaction from them about his being with you?"

"They didn't seem surprised, if that's what you mean. I told the wife I was a medical student working in the lab, and she thought it was nice more women were going to medical school. We didn't talk about whether he'd brought others to the opera."

"O.K. Go on."

"After the opera finished, his friends said goodbye, and Dr. Morris said he wanted something to eat. I told him I needed to get back, I had to study—at that point I just wanted the evening to end. He wouldn't take no for an answer—he did what he wanted. We went to a restaurant/bar sort of place, and he started drinking, you know, quick shots of vodka one after the other. He ordered dinner, I wasn't hungry. So I just sat there and watched him eat and drink. He seemed drunk; then he started talking about sex, and how much he enjoyed different women—that he usually preferred Orientals, because they're agreeable and have nice, straight silky hair." Her voice was breaking, and she looked directly at me. "You know, Dr. Conley, the technicians in the lab are all Asian!" She paused, then said, "He told me he thought I was somewhat exotic and that we could have a good time together. I kept begging him to please finish his food, I needed to get back, that I didn't want to hear any of this, that I wanted no part of it. Eventually, he staggered back to my car with me and I drove back from the city."

I was thinking my inclination would have been to leave him with his dinner and drinks and let the bugger find his own way back. But I knew, had I been Sonja, I probably would not have dared, not at that age and not at that stage in my medical education. My heart went out to her. She had to have asked herself many times that evening, "What in the hell am I doing here?"

But there was more.

"When we got to his house, there weren't any lights on. It was really dark because the driveway's off the street. As soon as I stopped the car he was all over me, pawing, kissing, trying to remove my clothes, begging me to love him. . . ." Sonja was now weeping openly. I offered her a small box of hospital Kleenex and she wiped her face and blew her nose. "I kept telling him over and over, 'No, no, this isn't right, I don't want this.' Finally I managed to get the door on his side opened, and shoved him out of my car onto the driveway and just drove off, leaving him sitting there. He was fairly drunk. . . ." After a couple more staccato sobs, Sonja regained control. "It probably wasn't right, but I kept working in that lab."

"Wait a minute," I interjected, "didn't you tell someone about all this?"

"Until today, my boyfriend is the only one who knows this happened—but it's ruined my life. I kept working in the lab, hoping he wouldn't really remember. I tried to set my hours so I wouldn't run into him, but one day he was there, much later than usual for him. He let me know 'nothing had happened that evening, understand?' But since the episode there'd been a subtle difference in the way I was treated by others in the lab. I was kind of shunned. The other faculty in the department had always been friendly and helpful, and now they were sort of avoiding me too, now that I think about it, and I began hearing rumors from others in the lab that I wasn't doing good work—wasn't smart enough. I knew why it was happening in the lab, but I kept on with my work, and finished what I thought was a good project. I'd done well on my clerkship in ophthalmology and gotten good evaluations from the residents, and I asked some of the faculty to write letters of recommendation for me. How was I to know they'd been brainwashed by Dr. Morris? I couldn't do anything. He controls them because he brings in money for them. Ophthalmology is a real small specialty. I'll bet I've been blackballed at every program in the country. I really don't know what to do . . ." Sonja was sobbing again.

I was crying with her. Sitting in front of me was someone whose life and career had been destroyed by hierarchical power and sexual harassment. I knew Sonja wasn't crazy—her story was intense, and ever so credible. Sonja was absolutely correct. She would never be an ophthalmologist. Duane Morris had been sexually attracted to Sonja; the practical impact of that attraction was obvious. Ultimately, whether or not she had accepted his advances, he had the power to totally destroy her career and her future, if he so chose.

Sonja and I spent the next half hour exploring various strategies. It was too late to influence this year's match for residency positions, and I was not optimistic she would have a better chance the following year. I did not have to tell her this experience would follow her forever. She was reluctant to report the episode because she feared increased retaliation and backlash. I asked, "Sonja, what if you're not the only one Duane Morris has ruined? My bet is this is SOP for him—he gets away with this time and time again because everyone's too afraid to speak up and put an end to his scuzzy behavior. How about the Asian lab technicians—who's protecting them? Do you really want to be a mere statistic in his repetitive crap?" She was angry enough to take up my challenge, and agreed to meet with the appropriate administrative official, Bob Cutler.

I found listening to these stories very painful. The women involved had been so badly wounded, leaving but a pathetic, emotional shell where once a strong personality had thrived. But I had little to offer women from other academic institutions or workplaces except a sympathetic ear and some very basic strategic planning. So often women who bring a complaint of discrimination or sexual harassment become so emotional about events, their presentation is less than rational, in fact often is hysterical. Then, in domino fashion, the original abuse is followed by skepticism, followed by retribution for making a fuss in the first place, followed by termination or ostracism because people do not believe the "mentally deranged" accuser. Many who called had passed the point of no return with their school or workplace, leaving legal action as their only viable recourse.

After the Hill-Thomas debate, lawyers developed increasing interest in hearing about gender discrimination and unfair termination cases. Plaintiff attorneys, however, have always been ambivalent about challenging universities. The academic cocoon accepts our gawky, caterpillar-like children into its protected embrace, promising them transfiguration into beautiful adult butterflies over four or more years. How can society ever question an establishment in which we place such a precious trust? Historically, because of its profound institutional strength and the revered esteem the academy enjoys in our society, legal judgments have tended to favor universities. Few of the women I talked to had realistically appraised how a legal fight would transform them as people and professionals, how it would affect their career options, and—especially for physicians—how it would replace their openness and potential for caregiving with cynicism, distrust, and paranoia. It was imperative for them to understand that their past loyalty to an institution was not likely to be repaid in kind. My message was blunt: "Either forget it or fight it," neither being an easy choice. For some the decision to forget brought double guilt—enduring the insult, and then not having sufficient fortitude to challenge it.

In addition to serving as a magnet for women with troubles, I received many public speaking invitations, especially after the Hill-Thomas event. Some were local, others across the country. My calendar filled rapidly into the middle of 1992, and engagements included three commencement addresses to be delivered in late May. Most talks were to academic and/or medical audiences, and from these numerous trips I learned that conditions at Stanford, far from being unique, were paradigmatic: unequal and abusive treatment of women was prevalent—ubiquitous—in the working environment of our profession.

Almost every medical school I visited had arranged for me to meet with a high-ranking administrator (all male, except one), followed later by a meeting with a small group of women faculty working on women's issues at their institution. The women would start our session by surreptitiously asking how I had found their dean, or president, or chancellor, or provost. I learned to give a neutral response. The stories would then come pouring out. Did I realize the dean himself was guilty of numerous affairs? Or the provost had failed to admonish male faculty for proven egregious behavior? Or their chancellor was outwardly very interested in discrimination issues, but, in fact, condoned and permitted discrimination at their institution? The women were being paid less, not given maternity leaves, found meetings scheduled by their departments were at times when they needed to deliver or pick up children from day care or school, were being asked to do an inordinate amount of clinical work rather than research, and were not being promoted in percentage numbers equivalent to their male peers.

At most schools I also met with groups of medical students, frequently over lunch or dinner. The students were not at all hesitant to share stories with me, knowing my general theme and why I was visiting. At the University of Michigan two women students, learning physical diagnosis by practicing on each other, discovered that the faculty physician assigned to them and another group of two male students had spent twice as much time with them, had himself done unnecessarily rough breast exams on both of them, and had spent only cursory, "laid-back" time with the two men.

At the University of West Virginia Medical School I had lunch with the students and house staff in general surgery. The very first question I was asked, after routine introductions, was, "How can a woman go into surgery if she wants to have a baby?" I asked my inquisitor how many children he had. "Four," he answered.

"Do you ever see them?"

"Not much."

"Then why did you have four kids if you were going into surgery?" He had no immediate answer. The session was acrimonious. Toward the end of the hour, the chairman strolled in to see how things were going. He was dressed in a plaid shirt and overalls and had a bandanna looped loosely around his neck—all his "good ol' red neck" costume lacked was a disheveled straw hat, a piece of straw picking at his teeth, and a bottle of whiskey. Maybe he always dresses that way when he has visitors. His manner, however, was very condescending and clearly communicated the message: "Lady, we here don't like you very much, and we're gonna make sure you don't like us much either."

In response to my editorial written half a year earlier, Adriane Fugh-Berman, M.D., wrote a blistering condemnation of Georgetown Medical School and her experiences there as a student.[1] One of many examples of sexism occurred in a class on human sexuality (coined "he-man sexuality" by the urology professor who taught it). A psychiatrist told the students that aggression is normal in sexual relations between a man and a woman (was he offering an apology for rape?), and inhibition of aggression in men can lead to impotence. Another memory she shared was of a female student watching a surgeon teaching a minor surgical procedure to a male student. When the procedure was finished, the surgeon handed his bloody gloves to her so she could discard them.

In 1996, at the University of Washington, medical students were using a 1985 anatomy textbook that still contained only a rudimentary description of the breast. Fortunately, they received a handout with a more accurate, detailed discussion.

Also in 1996, a University of Colorado M.D./Ph.D. student found herself being escorted back to her residence by the NIH program coordinator after a dinner meeting. He invited her to join him and share a hot tub at his facility. From the tone of the invitation, she told me, he was after only one thing. She declined his kind offer politely, kindly, but firmly, having been forewarned about his reputation. However, she remains apprehensive about her future, as he may well be in a position to counter her rebuff by limiting her access to research funding once she is in a position to establish her own laboratory.

I heard stories from medical students at Johns Hopkins, SUNY, the University of Florida, the University of Minnesota, Harvard, Loma Linda, UC Davis, UCLA, the University of Texas

1 A. Fugh-Berman, "Man to Man at Georgetown: Tales out of Medical School," *The Nation*, January 20, 1992.

(Houston), the University of Massachusetts, Tufts, the University of Utah, Washington University in St. Louis, Yale, the University of North Dakota, the University of British Columbia, the University of Pennsylvania, Rush University, UCSF, Mount Sinai, Wayne State University, the University of Virginia, Albany Medical College, the University of North Carolina, the University of Cincinnati, the University of Medicine and Dentistry of New Jersey, the University of Arizona, and NYU Medical Center. Their stories were no different than what I had heard at Stanford. Common to all of them was the fact that women *were* treated differently, and the male students who attended these sessions agreed.

From schools across the country women faculty had distressingly similar stories with only minor variations on the major theme. Some, however, were beginning to fight. Two female psychologists working in the Psychiatry Department at UCSF filed a legal challenge over discriminatory job changes and eventual termination after refusing sexual relations with a supervisor. Because their suit alleged "emotional distress" from their experiences, they were required to undergo a psychiatric evaluation by a psychiatrist chosen by the university. This reprehensible practice is actually quite common in harassment cases, and is used to demonstrate a plaintiff's mental derangement in a court of law at the time of trial. I believe that the use of psychiatry in workplace disputes is particularly common at research or medical institutions, which have staff or affiliated psychiatrists to whom troublemakers can readily be referred. Unlike other employers, medical and research institutions can call up an in-house doctor and say, "There's this crazy woman who thinks she's been harassed. We need you to take a look at her." The implication is "Look, fella, get us off the hook."

At UC Irvine, women faculty found almost none were being promoted to tenure, the percentage of women on the faculty had remained stagnant for the past ten years, women faculty uniformly were paid $4,000 to $16,000 less than men for doing the same job, and then they discovered the university administration had withheld the results of an adverse summary containing this data from them and the rest of the university system. Faculty women mounted an impressive newspaper campaign and an anesthesiologist filed suit over her tenure denial. In order to meet her legal expenses, she was forced to sell her home.[2]

Women at the University of Virginia had collected data documenting gender discrimination and unequal pay and gave me a copy of their confidential report (meant only for the eyes of the administration). In March 1992, the university system began "boosting the salaries of female professors to bring them in line with those of male counterparts. . . . One professor's salary was increased 40 percent, school officials said" (*San Francisco Chronicle*, March 18, 1992).

On my first few lecture trips I had been surprised to find academic women physicians outside of Stanford who understood unequivocally and accepted without challenge my message about the corrosive nature of sexist "micro inequities." But I rapidly learned they all knew what I was talking about from their own personal experience. The atmospheres I encountered were, for the most part, depressing. Hopelessness had replaced any semblance of happiness or joy in work for these women. They were tired, discouraged, and had open psychic wounds from repeated encounters with solid brick walls and glass ceilings.

The solution to the harassment/discrimination "problem" at most medical schools was to appoint a relatively low-level administrator (usually a woman) to be "sexual harassment coordinator," or "omsbudsperson." Very few of these had a direct reporting relationship to the top dog—president, dean, chancellor, provost. However, I discovered two exceptions: Merle Waxman at Yale and Mary Rowe at MIT. Both have direct access to their respective president's ear and a true commitment from those at the top to eliminate these societal diseases.

2 See *Los Angeles Times*, December 18, 1992; *Orange County Register*, December 18, 1992; *Irvine World News*, January 28, 1993, among others.

The pervasiveness of the gender discrimination issue for the medical profession is also reflected in the fact that I was asked to speak before a number of specialty groups at their national meetings—anesthesiologists, emergency medicine doctors, endocrinologists, ophthalmologists, general surgeons, orthopedists, radiologists, and doctors in family practice. Invitations were conspicuously absent from such groups as cardiovascular surgeons, thoracic surgeons, vascular surgeons, and cardiologists (all highly paid interventionists in fields where women members are rare). I also participated in workshops or gave lectures to groups representing the American College of Surgeons, the American Medical Association, American Women in Science, and the Association of American Medical Colleges. Discrimination and harassment are universally encountered in our profession.

I gathered a number of personal stories from women doctors and have learned that the few other women who are neurosurgeons across the country share a rich legacy of experience with me. It ranges from inexcusable verbal abuse to attempted rape by a department chair. Eight years ago, as a medical student interviewing for a residency position, one female neurosurgeon was asked by a prominent program director why he needed a woman in his program. After all, he told her, he already had a wife! Another was told she could enhance her chances of becoming a neurosurgeon by having a sex-change operation along with a brain transplant. As recently as 1993 another was asked if she was one of those "girls" who take three days off every month. At a cocktail reception during a national meeting in 1989, as I tried to disentangle myself from an effusive, clutching embrace by an inebriated well-known neurosurgeon, who insisted on calling me "kitten," both sleeves on the dress I was wearing were ripped almost completely off. Everyone laughed. A general surgeon was told by an internal medicine colleague that he would not refer cases to her because she was too pretty and might well suffer from PMS in the operating room to the detriment of good patient care.

I also spoke to a number of undergraduate groups at Stanford.

Many male students attended the dormitory sessions, some from sheer curiosity about this creature who had tarnished their school's reputation. Others participated willingly in discussions of gender roles, working couples, child care, a wife with a larger paycheck. I found many men who desired and expected a traditional wife, despite working and studying alongside very capable women at Stanford. The women, in general, planned on a career and children in that order. One freckle-faced young man with unkempt hair told me, "I don't mind living in a dirty house, so if she wants it clean, it's her responsibility." I gently reminded him women were becoming increasingly tolerant of dust bunnies also, and, with his attitude, his house would be one where he would not be comfortable entertaining his boss. It was disheartening to find so many men from this college generation unwilling to consider they might need to share routine household chores more equally with their future mates.

In general I enjoyed being on the lecture circuit. It was marvelous to get away from the medical school for a few days at a time, and the diversion gradually replaced my deep depression with a psychological state of quiet anxiety and anger. Except for my experience in West Virginia and with some medical societies, where the audience was composed largely of angry white males who had enjoyed a drink or two, I was always greeted enthusiastically, with compassion and warmth.

However, the Neurosurgery Department back at Stanford was anything but warm or compassionate. Since July my only departmental contact had been with dark offices and friendly janitors as I picked up mail long after closing hour. The only neurosurgical faculty I saw during the summer was Dr. Joe Andrus on days he worked at the VA. Joe and I are good friends. When I resigned Joe knew there was a good chance Gerry would be confirmed as chair in the future, and he performed a brilliant juggling act between the two of us, maintaining a neutral stance essential for his own survival.

But the impact of my actions resonated there despite my physical absence. One of many newspaper articles had mentioned my alienation from the staff, and spawned the following letter to me from Dr. Lee Stein's secretary, Pam Jensen. (Dr. Lee Stein is an associate professor on the clinical line.) Pam's letter was written just before Thanksgiving:

Dear Fran,

It would be unwise for me (they'd rip my face off) to openly express my support for you. I therefore have chosen to remain as neutral as I can. While most others here see black and white (you're black), I realize that there are other colors to the spectrum. Frankly, the dean seems to be the primary rat, for not checking out Gerry's qualifications and leadership abilities (or lack of them) more before he named him chairman, and then for not backing up his decision once he made it.

I greatly admire your guts for stooping down and swooping up that very lumpy rug and saying, "Look at all this dirt that's been swept under here!" and leaving that dirt uncovered. Your actions, by someone who is well respected and heard, have catalyzed the possibility for some very positive changes in the department (and the country and the world, oh-by-the-way). While the majority of the department are spending their best energies to deny the realities that lay before them and cover up that dirt (dirt? What dirt?), I have tried my best to casually walk by and (oops!) uncover that rug again (Hey, what's this? It's still dirt!), working within the framework of the department and trying not to make too many enemies in the process. Yes, I'm still looking elsewhere [for a job], but not without feeling I've also done my best to see if things can't change and to see if I can

*have any impact (which is difficult when you're a peon sec-
retary).*

*Thanks for getting things going. You have my support,
gratitude, and respect.*

Sincerely, Pam
(P.S. Please don't share this with anybody who matters.)

Unfortunately, the traitor got caught. Pam left the letter on
her computer, where it was discovered by another secretary, who
circulated it widely. Pam bore the consequences alone. Dr. Stein
remained silent, unwilling to give protection and support to a
woman who had been loyal to him and was an excellent employee. Pam put up with open departmental hostility for another
miserable month and a half, then found happiness in a job away
from Stanford.

After the visit from Sonja, I found a place at the medical school
where women faculty and students could go for help. During the
summer Dean Korn had established and promised funding for an
Office for Women in Medicine and the Medical Sciences. The
program became a reality during the fall quarter after he named
Dr. Margaret Billingham its first director. His choice had been
deliberate and crucial.

Margaret is a tenured professor of pathology and had been a
member of the faculty when Korn headed that department. They
had been colleagues for years. She is honest, forthright, and as
well respected for her science as her reserved English personality.
Dean Korn knew she was the perfect person to listen and soothe,
to deflect and dissuade; she was also someone who would not
disappoint him. He gave her no power, but issued a silent mandate that she was to get the gender issue out of his office—permanently. Margaret has experienced her share of inequality
during her professional career—in less pay, less secretarial help,
less office and laboratory space. She had been vocal about the

injustices, often writing long, detailed memos; but every time she had stopped short of revolutionary action. Assimilating abuse, for herself and others, became part of her persona—shaking her head of short, wavy hair in disappointment—but most days presenting a charming smile of acceptance as she carved an illustrious career for herself wrought by years of hard, lonely work.

As fall turned to winter and the investigative panel was still at work with the Silverberg case, both Margaret and I gradually realized that more than one complaint about discrimination was coming from a single department—radiology. By now I was well aware that my trouble with Gerry was but the tip of an iceberg: faculty women all over the medical school were not being treated fairly.

The department chair of radiology, Dr. Gary Glazer, quite young and administratively inexperienced, had implemented an ambitious recruiting scheme, working to attract new technical faculty—those interested more in the physics of radiology than in day-to-day clinical application of their specialty. Tenure-line appointments had become increasingly valuable in an era of marked fiscal constraint, and his dream empire depended on the availability of tenured slots to lure competitive intellectual brain-power to Stanford. Faculty slots are limited by the university pro-vost's office, so to bring new faculty in, faculty already occupying tenure-line positions had to go. The chosen method was to create a hostile, intimidating, and nonsupportive environment for those whose exit was desired, hoping they would get the message and leave under their own volition.

In the late fall I visited Margaret in her office to share infor-mation, and saw a paper tablet by her phone with angry word doodles on it. She had traced them over and over, creating thick, dark characters: "Why do women put up with this?" Seven women were on the radiology faculty when Dr. Glazer assumed the helm. None had tenure, but five were on a tenure-line track. One by one, three of them had navigated the labyrinthine hall-ways to Margaret's small second-floor office tucked out of sight in pathology, about as far from radiology as one can get. They told Margaret what was happening in their professional world. Dr. Glazer had taken their offices for male faculty he had just recruited, he had added his own name to their research grants, he did not allow them their fair share of research time, he had even stopped their access to patients whom they were following in clinical trials they had started prior to Glazer's arrival at Stanford.

For two years there had been unrest in the Radiology Department. Many male faculty were also markedly unhappy with Glazer's ruthless vendetta. One of the chair's prime targets had been Dr. Steven Yeager, a tenured associate professor who, in retaliation for what he saw as unfair practices, filed a formal grievance, claiming professional misconduct on the part of his chair. A hearing officer, a cardiologist, was appointed to investigate the charges. The formal grievance included reference to gender discrimination against female radiology faculty members. These were facts well known to both David Korn and Robert Cutler in late 1991 when Cutler's investigative panel was working on the Silverberg case. A pattern of institutional discrimination and attempts to hide it would become oppressively obvious in the future.

The end of the fall quarter at Stanford signals the end of the calendar year. All was quiet from the investigative panel. I figured they were going through some formal motions to generate something in writing to defuse any future legal challenge from me. After all, my attorney had thirty-seven damning letters in his possession which the panel had to address—and negate. My lack of optimism about their ultimate findings and how they would interpret them was reflected in the fact that books, files, journals, and the rest of the contents from my office remained at home. The Perlroth case also remained quiet and unresolved.

Then during the Christmas break I encountered Bob Cutler

and asked him idly, "How are things going?" I expected a casual, uninformative social reply. But he answered to the effect that I did not know the half of it—nurses were the ones who had really suffered.

I tried not to get excited, but this was valuable information. I asked how much longer the investigative effort would take. He said he didn't know. I continued. "I've not had the heart to keep working in my laboratory or finish up a grant application, and don't intend to do so until I know the outcome—I hate doing work that ultimately has no meaning." A grim smile passed his face, and without hesitation he told me I should re-up my lab, that I had nothing to worry about.

I could not help it now—I was elated. Maybe the situation was not hopeless after all. Our brief encounter told me at least some people had been willing to talk, and when they did, the panel was hearing what I thought they would hear. Although the panel report would be kept confidential and was subject to interpretation by Dean Korn, Bob's subtle news was gratifying. I know it is inappropriate to take solace in the travail of others, but I had been at war alone for six long months, acquiring along the way a harsh battle mentality infused with a strong dose of paranoia and vindictiveness.

Phil and I received our annual holiday greeting card from Dean Korn. One was mailed to every faculty member. This year the dean had chosen not to use automatic address labeling, and, in a nice touch, had commissioned someone to write on each envelope by hand. Our card was addressed to "Mr. and Dr. Philip Conley," despite Phil's never having obtained or desired a doctorate degree. In a flourish of beautifully scripted handwriting, my presence at the medical school had been eliminated—again. Phil said I was being petty.

As the new year started, Phil and I spent a few days watching seals and storm surf from the deck of our north coast house. I was fully aware 1992 might be just as negative and unhappy as 1991 had been.

11 Time was being used as a potent weapon as the first month of the new year slowly gave way to the second. I yearned for some type of resolution and closure. My life was on standby, and a cold-war climate prevailed between the medical school and me. Based on Cutler's brief remarks in December, I had let myself believe some type of action might be imminent. Thus I was loath to interfere and try to push things along, but found little energy to persevere against the unknown. Institutional administrators are familiar with this repetitive pattern, and find procrastination a friendly vice. With time, many vexing problems do disappear on their own, fading into the oblivious world of the "no longer important."

Then in the first two weeks of February a number of the dean's lingering problems began to surface. The hearing officer reviewing Dr. Steven Yeager's grievance from the Department of Radiology gave his report to Korn and Cutler. It supported the majority of Dr. Yeager's positions. His written report ended: "the grievance as a whole may be viewed as part of a still larger problem." The deans asked the hearing officer to modify his report to cast a more favorable light on Dr. Glazer. He refused.

On February 7 the *San Francisco Chronicle* ran a short article, unimpressively titled "Stanford Censures Professor." Heart pounding, I read the public statement released by the university: "Stanford University President Donald Kennedy announced that the professional misconduct charges brought against medical school professor Dr. Mark Perlroth have been formally resolved. The resolution includes disciplinary measures that are contained in a letter of censure—the text and terms of which will remain confidential. The details of the resolution have been reviewed and approved by the [two medical student] complainants. Dr. Perlroth wishes to apologize for his insensitivity and for his departure from appropriate hiring practices. . . . With the resolution Kennedy now has withdrawn the formal charges from the Advisory Board."

My Advisory Board colleagues had spent innumerable hours with hearing officers and attorneys, working through an arcane and incredibly cumbersome procedural disciplinary code, only to have the case settled, behind closed doors, in an agreement reached between Dr. Perlroth's attorney and the university counsel. Knowing I would be accused of conflict of interest, I had not participated in this Advisory Board activity.

Nine months had passed since I had heard the first rumblings about Dr. Perlroth at the Medical Faculty Senate meeting. It had been an even longer time between the filing of the original grievances by the two female students and the announced resolution. The sealed legal action precluded our university community from learning anything from the case about boundaries of acceptable behavior. In addition, it was impossible to ascertain whether the institutional response to recidivistic behavior had been sufficiently punitive to act as a deterrent against future harassing episodes. While discussing Perlroth, the university General Counsel said that in the twenty-three years he had been with Stanford, he had never heard of another case of sexual harassment charges being filed against a faculty member. As if no charges equaled no problems.

Also in early February, Dean Korn's secretary called with a sudden and unexpected invitation to meet with him that evening. It had been months since my last contact with Korn. I had little reason to expect favorable news. By report, Gerry was still acting cocky and self-assured. I told myself the report from Cutler's committee was probably in the dean's hands and he had decided it did not contain sufficiently damning evidence to require more than a figurative hand slap, if that. Furthermore, rumors were circulating that the dean's solution to the neurosurgery "mess" was to eliminate its departmental status and convert it into a division under the Department of Surgery. Such a move would eliminate any outside interest in a chair position; therefore, it would not be necessary to reopen a national search. Gerry could be maintained as divisional chair, certainly a demotion from a departmental chair position, but probably enough to repay an outstanding debt. I would be sufficiently unhappy about Gerry's continued control over my workplace that I would finally leave, this time for good. The media would be happy justice had been served. With the passage of yet more time, Dean Korn could again do exactly what he had intended in the first place.

The encounter that evening was brief and very strange. The dean quickly told me he had not yet been given the report. Then he surprised me by inquiring whether I was interested in heading up the newly created sports medicine program. From what I understood about the program, it was not Korn's prerogative to appoint its chief. Just as he had done with my VA laboratories, he was attempting to manipulate circumstances over which he had little control. What was he trying to wiggle out of this time? Over the past eight months I had acquired a healthy distrust for the man. I gave him a puzzled look and told him I would talk with others more knowledgeable than I about the pros and cons of the position, and get back to him.

I got up and walked to the door. My back was facing Korn when he suddenly said, "I hope you don't think I had anything to do with your labs, 'cause I didn't." I stared at him, looking over my shoulder, shaking my head in disbelief. Now he was openly lying. But I said nothing. I felt absolutely drained. The energy necessary to confront and contradict him just was not there. Two days later I talked with the architect of the sports medicine program, who confirmed that Korn was again giving away something he did not own. Was he making one final move to save the chair for Gerry? Or was he desperately trying to avoid a lawsuit in which he would be named a defendant—an event that now could be triggered by either of us? In any event, sports medicine was never a viable career option for me.

However, Sonja, the would-be ophthalmologist, found her life and career changed forever, and she felt powerless to stop it. She had met with Associate Dean Robert Cutler in January and found him not very helpful. He said he saw no way of intervening in the residency match on her behalf. Her only option, he had told her, was to file a grievance against Dr. Morris. He added that the grievance would go to the department chair for the first round of adjudication, and it would be her word against Morris's, because the alleged events happened in the absence of witnesses. Under those conditions both Sonja and Cutler knew she had little chance of emerging victorious. The chair of ophthalmology had a marked conflict of interest. A chair is expected to maintain a functional, productive unit, and to protect his faculty, not punish them. It would have been suicide for him to have gone after Duane Morris. Dr. Morris's power lay in his monetary value to the department. When handed a formal grievance, the natural inclination for a chair is to get it off the agenda rapidly, with as little threat to departmental stability as possible. If the miscreant is one of the good old boys, denial and cover-up is that much more expedient.

Every month the editorial staff and reporters of the *Peninsula Times Tribune* invited someone to meet with them for an off-the-cuff, off-the-record session at their headquarters. I was their guest for February 1992, and I shared Sonja's story with the group, using assumed names and not identifying the department. With my permission, but without identifying me in any way, one of the writers used the story as the basis for his weekly editorial, titled "Legacy of Sexism: Reform on the Surface Doesn't Preclude Bias." It relayed Sonja's story, anonymously and poignantly. The editorial ended with the sentence "All the institutional reforms and education and platitudes about equal opportunity are ultimately inadequate as long as outdated thinking is characteristic of those in power" (*Peninsula Times Tribune*, February 18, 1992).

The next day I got a summons to meet with Dr. Cutler and the other senior associate dean from Korn's office. They were furious. The two of them insisted I write a letter to the editor to correct a minor factual mistake the writer had made, and include the information that the dean's office had responded appropriately to Sonja and the harassment incident. They told me Sonja had not matched in ophthalmology because it was a highly competitive specialty, and she was just not quite good enough. Oh, really? I thought to myself—the real reason is that David Korn cannot tolerate having another accusation of sexual harassment at this school added to his agenda and will do almost anything to get rid of it. I was quite upset that the two associate deans had capitulated to Korn so readily. The report about Gerry had not yet been released and I did not want to ruffle Cutler's feathers unduly, so I placated them with a carefully worded letter (which was published). It concluded: "It is well known, however, that the intertwined nature of medical education within a hierarchical structure creates situations where a harasser has the opportunity to influence, for a lifetime, the career of those he or she chooses to harass. No matter what the facts are that led to failure of this student to match in her desired specialty, the failure would be easier to accept had the specter of harassment not been part of the scenario." (*Peninsula Times Tribune*, February 20, 1992).

But the damage had been done. Stanford Medical School won. Sonja was so intimidated by the strength of the fraternity and so fearful retribution would continue to haunt her life and career, she elected not to file a formal grievance. She changed her career plans, discarded her dreams of becoming an ophthalmologist, and entered a residency training program in physical medicine and rehabilitation.

David Korn received the Cutler report, a six-page confidential document about Gerald Silverberg, on February 13, 1992. I was not informed it had been completed. It was not until March 20, more than one month later, that an official announcement was made about its contents, and the university's response to it specified. Interestingly, portions of it were out in the open long before then and acted to defuse a more dramatic impact.

On Saturday, February 22, a front-page article in the *Peninsula Times Tribune* was titled "Demotion Is Latest Chapter in Stanford Med-School Flap." According to the article, Gerry announced he had been demoted because the university had "buckled under the media pressure." In a bizarre move, perhaps made to galvanize support and sympathy, perhaps in response to advice from his attorney to begin damage control, Gerry had contacted the press on Friday after a Wednesday afternoon meeting with Dean Korn and President Kennedy. Gerry was quoted as saying "he was demoted because the school has become very sensitive to media pressure and Dr. Conley had threatened to turn up the heat." He told reporters he had seen the confidential report and stated it detailed "minor insensitivities" on his part, but no "chargeable" offenses. He further informed them, "I don't believe anything in the report would hang anybody. I don't believe I've done anything wrong or different than any other chairman at the medical school. I understand where the school is coming from. They could no longer endure the adverse publicity."

It was the same type of argument Mark Perlroth had offered nine months earlier: had the media not interfered, there would have been no charges, no investigations, and no reprimands. Both men considered themselves victims of a system now operating under rules they had never encountered and did not understand. Neither apologized.

President Kennedy was asked to comment. He stated only, "What Professor Silverberg has announced is his own decision. It doesn't make a lot of sense to say the university has responded to pressure" (*Stanford Daily*, February 24, 1992). The only further information Kennedy provided was that their initial meeting was the first of several to be held between Gerry and his attorney and the university, and whatever had transpired at the meeting had been based on the Cutler report.

On Sunday morning the head of Stanford's News Bureau called me at home and asked if I had any comment about the evening news. "How can I comment when there's been no official announcement?" I said. "I don't even know if Silverberg's telling the truth. I'll wait until I see a statement from the university." In fact, I had no idea how to respond to the news report. The university's official action might, in actuality, be very different from Gerry's prediction, driven as it would have to be by legal constraints. I was cautiously optimistic, but remained wary.

On Monday a reporter from the *Stanford Daily* called, pleading for my reaction to the story. I love student reporters. They are so serious, so innocent. I told her I was shocked by Professor Silverberg's announcement of a demotion, and that if it proved true it would represent an unprecedented move by the university, one far in excess of what I expected or had even requested. All I had wanted was for the search to be reopened. Because Gerry had chosen to editorialize about the contents of the confidential report, I added that I thought the report should be released. Anonymity should be preserved for those who had provided information, but our community had the right to learn about behavior Gerry had characterized as "minor insensitivities."

As days went by and the university failed to confirm Gerry's demotion, it rapidly became a non-event.

On Thursday, March 19, Gerhard Casper of the University of Chicago was named the ninth president of Stanford University. The announcement was greeted by expected, and deserved, media attention.

In a carefully contrived timing maneuver, the medical school issued a press release about Gerald Silverberg the next day in the late afternoon, when media folk were exhausted from covering the new president. The release had been drafted at meetings with Gerry, Dean Korn, and attorneys representing Gerry and the university, and read in part:

> Vice President and Dean David Korn confirmed today that Dr. Gerald Silverberg will no longer be acting chairman of the Department of Neurosurgery, nor is he a current candidate for the chairmanship. Dr. Lee Stein has been named acting chair, effective March 20, 1992 . . .
>
> Korn confirmed that in a recent meeting, he and Kennedy "told Silverberg that they found certain behaviors described in the confidential [Cutler] report to be inconsistent with the leadership role of department chair. . . . We also told him we believed [these] behaviors reflected a troubling insensitivity, especially toward gender issues, and suggested that he make a serious commitment to correct this. He has accepted these suggestions, and I believe he made the right decision."
>
> Silverberg said that during the next year he has agreed to participate in training and counseling programs focused on gender insensitivity and that a procedure will be set up to review his behavior and monitor the work environment of the Department of Neurosurgery.
>
> "It is my hope," said Dr. Silverberg, "that this process

will lead to an improved, more communicative environment." Silverberg added, "I sincerely want to apologize to anyone I may have offended.

"It was never my intention to demean or insult any women, but it is now clear to me that some things I said or did in jest or from affection were taken as signs of disrespect.

"It is hard for me to accept this, but since I intend to make sure that my future actions do not give rise to such interpretations, I recognize that the first step towards this goal requires me to acknowledge that some of my behavior was offensive to others.

"I had a very emotional reaction to the report," Silverberg said. "I was amazed and distressed by it, particularly since some of the accounts it contained were from women whom I considered to be friends and hold in high regard, and whose professional abilities I greatly value. I regret that there were times when I didn't realize how I was coming across and hope they can believe that I didn't intend to insult or humiliate them."

Korn said that he was pleased by Professor Silverberg's plans. "I believe that with sufficient effort sexist and other forms of discriminatory behaviors and attitudes, even deeply ingrained attitudes, can be changed," Korn said. "That's what we are depending on as we work towards creating an environment free of sexual harassment and all forms of intimidation. . . ."

Korn said that at this point he was not prepared to speculate as to when a permanent department chair for neurosurgery might be appointed.

My name was conspicuously absent from the text. I was on the East Coast when the news was released, and had been given no advance warning. When I returned home Sunday, there were many phone calls and notes expressing congratulations. I had won, but at considerable cost. It all seemed quite anticlimactic.

Despite the attempt by the medical school to slip the story surreptitiously past members of the press, it attracted considerable media interest, with many headlines over the next days and weeks highlighting the "sensitivity training" Gerry had agreed to. No one knew what the "training" would consist of (neither did the medical school), but the thought was intriguing and tantalizing.

The Cutler report is, and remains, a confidential university document. I have never read it and do not know the identity of all those who were willing to talk. But if pseudonyms were used, I believe it would provide valuable education for all medical schools. Not only would it serve to refine the distinction between "sexual harassment" and "sexism" (genderism); it would also define acceptable and nonacceptable behavior (both verbal and physical) for our academic environment. I know Gerry is only one of many at Stanford who have exhibited behavioral irregularities. In order to truly change a culture, leadership roles must be denied to *all* who are "guilty."

I am not sure what David Korn thought Bob Cutler would find in the course of his investigation, or whether he expected Bob to operate as honestly and scrupulously as he did in gathering data. But in my opinion, Dean Korn was quite surprised when the investigative panel corroborated my allegations of nonsuitability for executive leadership. The sad truth is, I believe he thought women would maintain their traditional silence.

Thus the "heroine" of the "Conley story" is not Conley. There were approximately twenty "heroines," twenty "angels of mercy," mostly nurses, along with some clerical staff, who were willing to break a covenant of silence and tell the truth about unacceptable "flirtatious" behavior. The nurses defied the traditional doctor-nurse relationship in which the doctor is god, capable of no wrong, and the nurse his sweet, silent handmaiden.

The angels demonstrated extraordinary courage in telling the world about abusive behavior in the medical school, clinics, and hospital. Standing alone, I had looked like an embittered, opportunistic fool. But when others put their more vulnerable careers on the line to stand with me, suddenly I gained credibility.

A week after the official announcement, I met briefly with Dean Korn at his invitation. He asked me if Lee Stein was an acceptable acting chair. I answered, "Yes, he's a decent person—but the appointment shouldn't be forever."

With remarkable insensitivity and a hint of sarcasm Korn then said, "Well, things worked out the way you wanted, didn't they?" I was flabbergasted. Did he really think I was celebrating?

We were both standing by the circular table, his gaze fixed on the floor, mine on his downcast face. I reminded him there was still no national search for the chair position. He did not reply. Then, in a sudden overpowering wave of anger and profound, agonizing pain over my career that he had changed forever and essentially ruined, I said, "Don't ever underestimate me again, David." I paused for a long moment, trying, without success, to engage his eyes, then continued in a softer tone of voice, "And don't underestimate the power of the message your actions with regard to Gerry will deliver to this medical school, and maybe even to the rest of the medical profession. If you can break with your *own* internal bonds that tie *you* to inappropriate old-fashioned thinking and behavior, the school has a chance and you will have made a real difference." His face became an emotionless mask.

All of us in neurosurgery were wondering what it would take to function again as an integrated unit. What little optimism I had about an easy transition faded completely when I received a phone call from a fellow male neurosurgeon, a good friend on the East Coast, who had applied for the position as chair in early 1991. "What on earth's going on at Stanford?" he demanded. He had received a letter from Lance Dickenson, the neurology professor who had directed the search committee, informing him, "The search for a permanent chairman of the Department of Neurosurgery at Stanford University School of Medicine, which was temporarily suspended last year pending resolution of some internal issues, has been terminated and will not be reopened in the near future." David Korn had told Lance that no one would be interested in Stanford neurosurgery now, and, punitively, decided to relegate the department to its own internal purgatory. It was leaderless and dysfunctional and would remain so until the dean chose to act.

In April I met with Lee Stein and Bob Cutler to discuss the resumption of my clinical work at Stanford Medical Center. I told them I was willing to give it a try.

In May, Gerry had surgery on both eyes, leaving him temporarily without useful vision. He did not come to work, operate, or see patients for the next seven months. Also, any program of sensitivity training for him was placed on hold. With Gerry's absence my reintegration into the neurosurgical unit was actually somewhat easier than I had anticipated.

I began seeing patients, operating, and attending conferences at Stanford although the atmosphere with my colleagues was strained. Nurses on the floor and in the operating room, however, greeted my return enthusiastically and warmly. The OR nurses, in particular, had become empowered, and for the first time ever, I heard nurses berate surgeons about their behavior, saw challenge to unacceptable dialogue, and, in general, found decreased hierarchy in the surgical suite.

Dr. Kathy Purcell, the female resident who had joined our program in 1988, was now three years from finishing. She had been with me at the VA when I resigned, but had been back at Stanford since and was weathering the turbulence in our department quite well. Gerry had treated her with kindness, as well as carefully, knowing he was under scrutiny, and she, and her career, benefited greatly from his friendship, mentoring, and teaching. At the first conference I attended I was sitting alone in a classroom with many more seats than occupants. As others had come into the room, they had glanced at me, then looked again, with some disbelief that I was actually there. I was left sitting by myself. When Kathy came in, shortly after the conference started, she looked around, saw me, and, without a word, but with a big, bright smile, took the seat next to me.

With Gerald Silverberg's demotion, the atmosphere at the medical school turned sunshine bright and full of hope for women who worked there. We thought our school would assume a leadership position in directing a culture shift within the medical field. As director of the program of Women in Medicine, Professor Margaret Billingham felt she had an unmet obligation to tackle the troubling series of incidents which were occurring in radiology. Finally, now, she thought, there would be a receptive audience in the dean's office interested in addressing the issues and changing things.

Margaret visited Bob Cutler first, because she knew he was painfully aware there were significant problems. Cutler surprised her by telling her that for him to do anything, he would require facts, numbers, and documentation of discrete incidents of harassment or discrimination. Without concrete data, he could not help. Unfortunately, history seemed to be repeating itself.

Margaret, focused and tenacious, decided to obtain the "concrete evidence" Cutler required, and began interviewing members of the Radiology Department, staff as well as faculty, men as well as women. She was convinced that "gender issues" would not go away by themselves, and equally determined not to let them be buried. She collated her findings and wrote a confidential letter, dated May 26, 1992, to Dean Cutler. The anonymity of those she had interviewed was protected as she had promised. According to her letter: "It is apparent the chairman is totally focused on his own interests and goals to put himself on the map at all costs, including overriding and ignoring all the rules of fairness, decency, responsibility to his staff, honesty, and gender discrimination to meet his own ends." Dr. Billingham also found "the young male cadre have apparently become worse in their attitude towards women because they are presumably following the role model of the chairman." She ended her letter, "If this matter is not looked into further and redressed expeditiously, I cannot bring myself to believe the medical school administration is serious in its attempt to combat gender discrimination. If the situation in radiology, which involves many women, is not corrected with real action, then I believe our system is one of platitudes and, unless support comes from the top, regardless of the value of the individual concerned, the atmosphere will remain unchanged because this sends the message that if you are valuable you can behave as you like. This is the situation in radiology at this time."

On June 7, the *San Jose Mercury News* ran a front-page article, "Medical School Sexism Revisited." A year and five days had passed since the first article about me had been published. Somehow the contents of Margaret's confidential letter had been leaked to the press.

Deans Korn and Cutler were furious and not about to lose again. A protective wall was instantaneously erected around Dr. Glazer. Then the messenger was shot. As it turned out, a brutal process of threat and intimidation had been well underway even before the letter was leaked. Bob Cutler sent a terse memo to Margaret on May 29 accusing her of personally charging the chair of radiology with professional misconduct. A few days later she was asked to meet informally with Cutler, and walked, without warning, into an interrogation session complete with a court reporter. Dr. Glazer threatened her with a lawsuit for libel. So by the time the media had been summoned, fear had silenced Margaret. Both Korn and Cutler openly and vehemently denied having prior knowledge about problems in radiology, despite considerable evidence to the contrary—Dr. Steven Yeager's grievance papers and the hearing officer's report.

Yet another investigative panel was created by Dean Korn to explore these new allegations of gender discrimination. This time, however, the panel was stacked in the dean's favor. Bob Cutler chaired it, and along with the other senior associate dean, there was a professor of pediatrics who was being considered for department chair, and Alison Stone, who had served on the Silverberg panel. Questions were raised about the neutrality of such a panel, so a staff woman on temporary leave, whose employment status had yet to be negotiated, was added. It was obvious to most people this panel was not nearly as interested in ferreting out the truth as it was in damage control.

There followed five months of fact finding. On November 3, 1992, election day, the medical school issued a carefully timed press release late in the afternoon titled "Faculty Committee Finds No Evidence of Gender Discrimination in the Radiology Department." Portions of the release read, "The women faculty and staff told the committee their complaints had been overstated, generalized, and inappropriately categorized as gender-related. Billingham's original perception of gender discrimination was caused in part by miscommunication, rumor, and innuendo. There had been no radiology faculty discussion or clear statements from the departmental leadership [about gender discrimination]. The reason: 'We didn't have the problem.' "

The report was received by women faculty at the medical school with a massive uproar heard only behind closed doors. Given the stories I had heard over many months, I was astonished by the findings—but at the same time I expected them. Dean Korn could not afford even a hint of another sexism scandal. The report insinuated that Margaret Billingham was a hysterical woman. Faculty women knew better. Clearly, congratulations I had received for changing the climate at our school had been ridiculously premature. There was now backlash, and probably we should have been smart enough to expect it. The dean's position of total denial about any wrongdoing in radiology was vicious, carefully contrived, and highly effective. There could not have been discrimination, the report claimed, because both men and women in the department had been affected.

Over the next seven months, five of the seven female faculty from radiology left Stanford Medical School to accept positions elsewhere. None was recruited away—the women themselves sought relief from a harsh, hostile work environment. Some male faculty, including Dr. Steven Yeager, also relocated or took early retirement, but the percentage loss between the genders was nowhere near equivalent.

In December 1992 the EEOC attorney called to say the Washington office had not approved the request from San Francisco to start a class action suit against the university. He told me he was very surprised because they had gathered an amazing amount of evidence and information. He finished the conversation by saying, "Stanford has powerful friends in very high places."

But Pandora's box had been opened during the neurosurgery investigation, and Stanford had no way of shutting its lid. Abuses continued, as did the cries for help.

In March 1993, I met Helen Bae, a research assistant with plans to go to medical school. Helen is Asian-American, full of life and bubbly charm. She was working for Dr. Seymour Levine, an internationally known research scientist in the Department of Psychiatry at Stanford. She asked me how she could stop the hugging and kissing he forced on her. Her boss's excuse for his actions was that he could not help himself—that he was just a friendly "teddy bear" kind of guy.

But his behavior in the laboratory was not limited to the occasional hug or illicit kiss. Dr. Levine also talked openly about his sexual proclivities and his willingness to donate sperm. He unhesitatingly articulated his desire to sleep with his workers. In one episode, he leered at Helen and told her he would do what his dog, Opus, does, and grabbed Helen's head and licked and slobbered on her nose with his tongue. Helen privately asked Dr. Levine to stop his disgusting behavior, after which he began berating her in front of the whole group about her "goddamned feminism and assertiveness." He threatened Helen: that she would not gain admission to medical school without a favorable letter of recommendation from him. Before visiting me, Helen had met with Bob Cutler. He told her she had two options: quit her job or file a grievance. No effort was made to transfer her to another workplace or to stop Dr. Levine's objectionable behavior. Cutler also warned Helen to have no contact with Margaret Billingham or me.

The hostility between Helen and Dr. Levine escalated. He made an early morning menacing phone call to Helen's home. She was sufficiently frightened by his behavior that she quit. Then she filed a formal grievance, and once more the situation was investigated by three members of the medical school faculty chosen by Dean Korn. During the course of the investigation, Helen's boyfriend was asked whether she wore tight and revealing clothes to work. Her co-workers, badly frightened by Levine and the investigative process, verified Helen's claims but said that "Levine was just being Levine" and meant no harm.

In January 1994, eight months after the grievance was filed, the university found Professor Levine guilty of "professional misconduct," the by now familiar university catchall phrase. The only action taken was to place a letter of censure in his personnel file and to arrange for an occasional, unannounced visit by a monitor to his laboratory. Helen was told Stanford had chosen not to dismiss or suspend Levine or to reduce his pay, because "so many people depend on him" (he had a large research grant). Drs. Korn and Cutler, along with President Gerhard Casper, had managed to dispense with a case of sexual harassment in the medical school without any fanfare whatever—or so they thought.

232

Three months later, in April 1994, Helen broke into the secret world of university cover-up. With the help of a female professor of psychiatry who in 1977 had been an assistant professor without tenure working under Professor Levine, Helen unearthed a horrifying story of sexual harassment, intimidation, and retribution by the professor against four female employees in his research group. The abuses had been carefully chronicled and revealed to administrative sources seventeen years earlier. Dusty, forgotten files regurgitated compelling written testimony about past events, catapulting them into present real time.

I received an unsolicited letter from a woman who had been a graduate student in Levine's laboratory in 1976. It described the professor's past behavior, as well as its subsequent impact on the student's professional life: "In his office for the second time to discuss the research results, he suddenly unzipped his pants and pulled out his penis. He came forward and put his hands down the back of my hands, pulling me toward his crotch. I was completely shocked. I felt like a deer paralyzed by oncoming headlights. I couldn't react or move. I felt as though I would be killed, as if someone had just run over me with a semi. Somehow I got out of there. What he did to me had such a devastating impact, I shortly dropped out of school. It took many years to restore my equilibrium, my sense of psychological and physical boundaries, my self-esteem and respect."

The provost of the university at the time had written a confidential letter of censure and attached it to Dr. Levine's personnel file. It clearly documented his excessively familiar behavior with female staff. It stated Seymour Levine recognized the inappropriate nature of his actions, and gave "personal assurances that there would be no repetition of such behavior." The provost ended his letter, "[I] am putting it on the record here because, in event of recurrence, it is important to note that this has been discussed and that Professor Seymour Levine has been warned that such behavior is unacceptable." David Korn, Robert Cutler, and Ger-

hard Casper had all read the former provost's letter before deciding on the severity of sanctions to be levied against Levine in
January 1994.

I was outraged. I finally accepted the harsh reality that the
university leadership had learned absolutely nothing from their
recent experience, and would continue to play the cover-up game
if they could get away with it. I met with Helen's attorney and
encouraged her to file a lawsuit, despite knowing it would be a
tough battle. If any plaintiff could win in a court of law against
a university, Helen was that plaintiff.

The lawsuit was filed against Stanford University in May
1994. Levine, Cutler, Korn, and Casper were named as defendants. The suit alleged the university had failed to respond adequately to the documented harassment. We all knew many
months would elapse before the case would come to trial or
would be settled. Helen was short of money because of legal fees,
and faculty women established a fund to help her.

On August 24, 1994, catching many of us by surprise, President
Casper asked for David Korn's resignation, effective in one year.
I was overjoyed—Casper was finally acting to eliminate someone
who, in recent times, had not served the medical school well. In
his public statements Casper simply said that a new era of health
care demanded new leadership. Korn told the press he was being
forced out. The full inside story has never been released. But a
university spokesman was quoted as saying, "Korn's departure
has nothing to do with the sexual harassment controversies that
have bedeviled the medical school in the past few years." That
evening the Conleys shared a bottle of champagne.

At the end of August, I joined Professor David Kuechle at
Harvard University for an executive education program, concen-
trating on crisis management. We discussed the "Conley case"
with a group of university attorneys and also told them about
Dean Korn's forced resignation a few days before. At the end of

the session one of the attorneys raised his hand. He looked directly at me and said, "If I'd been advising your dean, I'd have told him in 1991, during that summer, no matter what happens—press or no press, lawsuit or not—don't ever let her come back on the faculty."

In October 1994, after more than four years of a highly publicized federal investigation, President Casper announced resolution of the government's indirect-cost dispute with Stanford. All claims that the university had overbilled the government by $200 million in research costs were dropped in exchange for a $1.2 million fee. The rate at which indirect costs could be recovered, however, remained much lower than it had been prior to the accusations. So the university's daily cash-flow problems continued.

Dr. Thomas Stamey, chair of the Department of Urology, was relieved of his executive position by President Casper in November 1994. This settled a grievance brought by a female staff member alleging sexual harassment. Financial sanctions were also levied against the professor. Publicly he denied the charges. Close associates told me he had exposed himself to a few women, but had done so in a "teaching" context and never intended any harm or harassment by his actions.

On April 6, 1995, five days after Dr. Eugene Bauer, formerly chair of the Department of Dermatology, was named as the new medical school dean, I attended a dinner with a small number of university colleagues. As we sat down to dinner, the Helen Bae–Seymour Levine legal case became the topic of discussion. I was surprised; it had not yet gone to trial or been settled. Usually active cases against a university are off limits as subjects for casual conversation. One of my friends, ostensibly knowledgeable about the case, said he really didn't understand what they were after—that they wanted to sue just because the offense had been labeled "professional misconduct" and not "sexual harassment."

I replied, "You must be joking! Is that what the university counsel is saying? Surely you don't believe that." A glass of wine had loosened my tongue, but not yet dulled my thinking. "Helen filed suit because the university did nothing to stop repetitive sexually harassing behavior. Seymour Levine has a past history the dean and president knew about, and yet all they did was to place another letter of censure in his file—big f—ing deal, pardon my language, but he thinks he's entitled to whatever he wants, and all they've done is to make the game more exciting for him."

"But it's been seventeen years between complaints!"

"And you believe nothing has happened in that laboratory during that seventeen-year period?"

"There is no proof that there was any misbehavior."

Another colleague broke in, also directing his comment to me. "You always seem to get very bothered when this sort of thing is discussed. Why is it so important to you?"

After I took a deep breath to control increasing anger, my brief response went to a larger group. "Because the woman's life is ruined, her professional career is derailed, or even abandoned, and no one with any power to change things cares. All of you in academics regard harassment or discrimination as a peccadillo— wrong, but not serious enough to jeopardize a *man's* career. What about the *women*?" There was a heavy, awkward pause and the conversation quickly moved to less contentious subjects. The evening ended in friendship and conviviality.

This snippet of conversation retains crystal clarity in my mind. The dinner, however, was not the time or the place to explode further, giving vent to my total frustration and genuine rage when trying to open people's eyes and change their minds and attitudes. My dinner companions themselves were unconscious icons of institutionalized sexism.

Three weeks later, Helen's lawsuit was settled out of court, almost a year after it had been filed. The settlement included payment of an undisclosed but substantial amount of money to Helen, letters of apology to her from all of the named defendants, and, in recognition that his actions might have adversely influenced her future career, a positive letter of recommendation from Levine about her professional ability as a research scientist. His laboratory was quietly closed and he was retired from the faculty.

When his sight recovered, Gerry returned to his full-time practice of neurosurgery almost as if nothing had happened. He never participated in a formal program of sensitivity training, although he had some sessions with a psychologist, a few of which I attended with him at his invitation. At these meetings he exhibited no interest whatever in modifying his behavior but was very intent on damage control. For example, he tried to extract a promise that I would stop all public speaking! "Honey" has a more limited place in his workplace vocabulary, but he has not yet mastered complete control over his mouth. He remains unnecessarily and harshly critical, and his negative comments continue to embellish our workplace. When we encounter each other I go out of my way to greet him with a cheery "Good morning, Gerry" and receive only a silent, vacuous, arrogant gaze in return. Abortive attempts were made through departmental staff-faculty-nurses meetings to address our hospital and clinic work environments, to institute behavior modification, and to raise the level of sensitivity to the feelings of others, all without appreciable benefit. Gerry has never forgiven or forgotten the nurses who were willing to talk to the panel—he maintains an icy aloofness with them, never asking "please," extending a "thank you," or even acknowledging their presence. Clinic secretaries and managers, who have been hired more recently, seem to have discovered a revolving door. Those who have left wonder why they stayed as long as they did.

A legitimate, open national search for a chair for my department never happened. For six years we were without permanent leadership, and Dr. Stein remained the acting chair. In December 1995, Dean Bauer named one of our associate professors (who won early promotion to full professor a few months later) to the chair position. The good news is the department now has someone with formal clout to fight for much needed renovation of clinic and laboratory space. The bad news is the person chosen was the former neurosurgical resident who, in 1986, allegedly made an uninvited evening visit to the home of a laboratory technician. I believe the technician's story. At the time she had nothing to gain and everything to lose by making an issue of Dr. Gordon Schloss's behavior. And she did lose everything—her job, her self-confidence, and professional respect. It has been ten years since the incident—have there been other episodes? Not to my knowledge. But sexism is alive in my department and at this medical school, and its legacy has been passed, with the mantle of power, to another generation.

I received over a thousand letters following my resignation. One was from Delaware, written in penciled block print. It read: "Dear Dr. Conley. My name is Mary Clare and I'm 12 years old. I hope to attend Harvard and be a pediatrician, however, I'm not sure now. I was upset after reading the article about you in the newspaper. Do you think my aspirations should be in the medical field? My aunt lives near San Diego, and if we ever visit California I'd like to meet you."

I do not know how I should answer Mary Clare. By the time she, but more probably her daughter, enters medical school, she might find the Stanford motto applies equally to everyone: "The wind of freedom blows—Die Luft der Freiheit weht." However, we academic women know we still face a major, uphill battle to make it happen.

AFTERWORD

A couple of years ago Gerald Silverberg was elected into the most prestigious and exclusive society of academic neurosurgeons—membership is politically determined but is usually reserved for those who are department chairs. At about the same time, in 1995, Dr. Thomas Stamey received the Achievement in Medicine annual award from the Santa Clara County Medical Association. Deviant behavior has never been a factor with sufficient strength to unravel the sturdy knots that twine the good old boys together, and, in fact, acts to coalesce their camaraderie, as I discovered so many years ago amid a pile of broken restaurant crockery. The status quo is maintained at almost any cost, including lying, cover-up, secrecy, and deceit when needed. It has always been the backbone of academic medicine, and to date, external forces have not been powerful enough to overthrow it.

In my "crusade" I dared those who enjoyed and benefited from the status quo to justify their God-given rights, and in so doing questioned the basic essence of a value system. It is a system white males were born into and which they thought would always be there for them. Unfortunately for all of us, it is a system predicated not only on the basis of capability but also on the basis of skin color and gender. When privilege diminishes, backlash kicks in as those facing a loss of *their* world as they know it make a desperate attempt to reestablish the status quo that supports their core values. "Diversity" has become a nasty word, and the molten lava of racism, never far from the surface, erupts again and again. Increasingly, we find the "have-nots"—women (especially those single and with children), minorities, the poor—trapped together in a common quagmire, marginalized, and served up as convenient scapegoats for those with power to decide how our society should look.

I have learned that universities, in general, no longer function as agents of societal change, as they did in my father's generation. The academic environment has become too imperious, too arrogant, too complacent, to be sufficiently introspective to observe and correct its own faults, let alone those of our society. Evolution within academia has made it dependent on outsiders with power—e.g., industry and wealthy alumni donors. Its liberal environment is a masquerade; in fact, academic centers are suffocating under a heavy cloak of unspoken conservatism, and increasingly are unwilling to accept any risk. Universities take inordinate pride in holding themselves out as enlightened places that create and respond to change, places that disseminate absolute truth and the most up-to-date research. However, they also possess all the foibles of institutions. Currently, their real desire is to maintain a comfortable status quo, exuding peace and tranquillity especially for the benefit of the press. Because vexatious issues rarely are allowed to surface, and in fact find a comfortable underground burrow, an amazing tolerance for behavioral irregularities has developed in universities. Stanford's medical school remains one such old-fashioned man's world. It is true that in my one brief skirmish with it, the "system" worked for me—but only because it was prodded by a tenacious media and presented with incontrovertible evidence. Even then, there was no revolution—not even reform.

The academic community has shown little inclination to change "business as usual," especially in adapting its structure to accommodate known biological differences in order to embrace the intellectual power of smart, ambitious, multitalented women who also want a family. Academia continues to use motherhood to massacre female possibility—requirements to do both jobs well are just too onerous, and lifestyle conflicts are almost inevitable. I was taught early in my life that a "woman's place was in the home," and have heard ever since (as a guilt trip) that women with careers upset traditional family stability—emotionally, economically, and socially. We now provide higher education for almost equal numbers of men and women, but equality for women who choose a career once they finish their education frequently is a myth. They, and usually not their mates, are the ones left with the hard choice. So many men in the medical profession, without really thinking about it and without adverse effect on *their* careers, marry early, raise a family in absentia, then divorce the first wife and marry again, this time a younger woman. Frequently they raise a second family (most have the economic means to do so), and this time the doctor gets involved and discovers the magic of life's meaning through his younger children. All of us should work to make this happen "right" the first time. But until we can view a man's willingness to help around the house and with his children as a necessity, rather than as a sublime gift of generosity, many husbands and wives will grow at disparate rates and in different directions, equality at home and/ or at work will remain a fantasy, and the divorce rate, at least among medical professionals, will continue to be high.

My concern was over the right leadership qualities and the potential they have to change our work environment for the betterment of all. I am no heroine. I would never have challenged Gerry or raised the specter of ubiquitous sexism in the medical environment had it not been for Gerry's appointment to department chair. With that move, Dean David Korn validated not only Gerry's behavior but also an old-fashioned template for success in academic medicine. However, I believe that inspired, progressive leadership by those with sufficient self-assurance and internal ego strength to make the necessary changes can alter the academic world sufficiently so that it regains its legitimate place in the next century. Unfortunately, as a country we have not demanded high ethical and moral standards for our elected leadership let alone those chosen within the academic arena.

The way leaders are selected in academic medicine is wrong. It favors those who have built their careers by intimidation and fear. Candidates for department chairs and deans submit a curriculum vita, give a seminar or grand rounds, interview with a few faculty, and are promoted on the basis of a written record of academic achievement, one or two days of sociability, and on the basis of who knows whom. No one bothers to call the head nurse of the operating room or the other "little people" at the candidate's present institution to inquire whether or not the staff enjoys working with him or her, whether or not he or she treats subordinates fairly, whether or not a passion for developing the careers of others has been evident. We tend to forget that love and respect can also confer immense power. When it comes to academic medicine, emotion, warmth, demonstrable humanity often are equated with weakness. Because these are so-called feminine traits, why should they be used as criteria when choosing a leader in a masculine-dominated culture?

On a personal level I have learned to get through one day at a time. I still work at Stanford although it is not always comfortable. I enjoy my time at the VA, which since 1975 has been my haven. I have been and still am a capable neurosurgeon. Respect and gratitude come from many patients I have cared for over a number of years, and I experience tremendous power as the result of my professional competence. But I now know I will never truly belong. This has been my greatest disappointment. One could ask why anyone would want to belong to this macho and, at times, not very attractive world. I believe there is a basic desire to establish deep, meaningful human contact through shared endeavors—an arduous training program, attainment of a high level of technical proficiency, a lifestyle of constant interruption, the angst and ecstasy that come from caring for those who are suffering. I worked as hard as anyone else, experienced all the incredible highs as well as the devastating lows my profession offers, and really thought I would make it and be accepted to full membership.

In addition, sixteen years of my professional life were negated when Dean David Korn callously tried to give away my laboratories. I have been unable to rekindle the passion I once had for scientific investigation. Running a research laboratory is an all-consuming endeavor, and with a thriving and increasing clinical practice, along with a heavy travel/lecture schedule, I found insufficient quality time or the requisite energy to devote to the research that once had been such fun. It also has been very painful to consider starting again since the work I did meant virtually nothing to those who should have appreciated it. Hopefully other scientists will continue our nascent work and discover the ultimate cure for malignant brain tumors.

"Was it worth it?" "Would I do it again?" The answer to both questions is a qualified "yes." At the time I had no choice—without action, my academic career at Stanford was essentially over. In many ways I have benefited greatly from my experience. The door to my cloistered, focused, noncreative cage was opened and I flew out into a big, wide, wonderful sky. I learned lessons not taught in books, expanded my horizons in directions I had no idea existed, met people I never would have otherwise, and have become both more and less tolerant about events in my external world. I suffer boredom less well, but also feel less guilty if my workday is less than twelve hours long. In 1992 I made a conscious decision to devote my few idle hours to reading good books, listening to good music, and living life. Thus I have reached a more refined balance between life's work and life's play, and enjoy small events, tiny observations, minuscule pleasures with greater intensity than ever before. My time with Phil— hiking, running, swimming, javelin throwing, philosophizing, sipping wine or downing shots of ice-cold vodka—has greater value and enjoyment.

A strange freedom comes from knowing that I have little to lose by telling this story. I have acquired a curious inner peace even realizing, in my lifetime, I will not see women obtain the equality of opportunity that should be theirs. Mine was but one battle, I was but one woman, Stanford was only one institution. But because of events of 1991–92 at Stanford, skepticism and cynicism have replaced complacent acquiescence and women now watch the entire landscape with increased acuity. So I can derive some comfort in knowing that my story is owned by a multitude of career women and some of them will continue its telling. And progress in that narrative will come from women who recognize and capitalize on the power that comes from coalitions and alliances with each other as well as with sympathetic men who believe in true equality. Only with a collective movement can women empower themselves to change the future for all of us. I at least tried, and thus face my own future with a great deal of equanimity. The beauty of every morning has returned to my beloved hills, and I have even learned to laugh again.

In mid-1997 I was promoted to the position of Acting Chief of Staff (initially these are almost always temporary appointments but many become permanent) at Palo Alto Veterans Health Care System, with responsibility over medical, dental, nursing, and paraprofessional staffs at three hospitals and three additional outreach clinics. I will continue to do a few neurosurgical cases, so my expertise as a highly trained surgical specialist will not be wasted. Within days of the Chief of Staff announcement, I was also elected chair of the University Senate (not the smaller medical school body)—the faculty forum for all of the schools of the entire university. Have I, and the stance I took, been vindicated at long last? Not really. I would much rather consider these posi-